ESSAYS IN BIOCHEMISTRY

Other recent titles in the Essays in Biochemistry series:

Lysine-Based Post-Translational Modification of Proteins: volume 52
edited by I. Scott
2012
ISBN 978 1 85578 185 6

Molecular Parasitology: volume 51
edited by R. Docampo
2011
ISBN 978 1 85578 184 9

ABC Transporters: volume 50
edited by F.J. Sharom
2011
ISBN 978 1 85578 181 8

Chronobiology: volume 49
edited by H.D. Piggins and C. Guilding
2011
ISBN 978 1 85578 180 1

Epigenetics, Disease and Behaviour: volume 48
edited by H.J. Lipps, J. Postberg and D.A. Jackson
2010
ISBN 978 1 85578 179 5

Mitochondrial Function: volume 47
edited by G.C. Brown and M.P. Murphy
2010
ISBN 978 1 85578 178 8

The Polyamines: Small Molecules in the 'Omics' Era: volume 46
edited by H.M. Wallace
2009
ISBN 978 1 85578 175 7

ESSAYS IN BIOCHEMISTRY

volume 53 2012

Cell Polarity and Cancer

Edited by Andrew D. Chalmers and Paul Whitley

portlandpresslimited
publishing innovation

Essays in Biochemistry is published by Portland Press Limited on behalf of the Biochemical Society

Portland Press Limited
Third Floor, Charles Darwin House
12 Roger Street
London WC1N 2JU
U.K.
Tel: +44 (0)20 7685 2410
Fax: +44 (0)20 7685 2469
email: editorial@portlandpress.com
www.portlandpress.com

British Library Cataloguing-in-Publication Data
A catalogue record for this book is available from the British Library
ISBN   978-1-85578-189-4
ISSN (print)   0071 1365
ISSN (online)   1744 1358

Typeset by Techset Composition Ltd, Salisbury, U.K.
Printed in Great Britain by Cambrian Printers Ltd, Aberystwyth

Contents

1 Cell polarity and asymmetric cell division: the C. elegans early embryo

Anna Noatynska and Monica Gotta

2 Phosphoinositide lipids and cell polarity: linking the plasma membrane to the cytocortex

Michael P. Krahn and Andreas Wodarz

3 **The role of secretory and endocytic pathways in the maintenance of cell polarity**

Su Fen Ang and Heike Fölsch

4 **Continuous endocytic recycling of tight junction proteins: how and why?**

Andrew D. Chalmers and Paul Whitley

5 **Crucial polarity regulators in axon specification**

Giovanna Lalli

6   Cell wars: regulation of cell survival and proliferation by cell competition

Silvia Vivarelli, Laura Wagstaff and Eugenia Piddini

7   The control of gene expression and cell proliferation by the epithelial apical junctional complex

Domenica Spadaro, Rocio Tapia, Pamela Pulimeno and Sandra Citi

8 Apicobasal polarity and cell proliferation during development

Nitin Sabherwal and Nancy Papalopulu

9 The Hippo pathway: key interaction and catalytic domains in organ growth control, stem cell self-renewal and tissue regeneration

Claire Cherrett, Makoto Furutani-Seiki and Stefan Bagby

10 Epithelial cell polarity: what flies can teach us about cancer

Daniel T. Bergstralh and Daniel St Johnston

11   The Scribble–Dlg–Lgl polarity module in development and cancer: from flies to man

*Imogen Elsum, Laura Yates, Patrick O. Humbert
and Helena E. Richardson*

Preface

The majority of cells exhibit some form of polarization by having an asymmetric distribution of macromolecules within them. This asymmetry is essential for important cellular processes including cell migration, asymmetric cell division and embryonic development. Epithelial cells have an extreme form of polarized morphology with distinct apical and basolateral plasma membrane domains. These cells also contain a number of specialized cell–cell junctions, including the tight junctions which are formed at the border between apical and basolateral membrane domains.

Polarized epithelial cells give rise to carcinomas that are responsible for approximately 80% of human cancers, and loss of epithelial polarity and junctions are thought to be key drivers in the process of tumour formation. There is currently great progress being made in understanding the establishment and maintenance of cell polarity, and how defects in polarity contribute to tumorigenesis. The present volume focuses on these areas and can be split into two overlapping sections: Chapters 1–5 focus on the establishment and maintenance of cell polarity, whereas Chapters 6–11 continue to consider the regulation of polarity, but have a greater emphasis on the links between polarity, tissue growth and cancer.

The first section starts with Chapter 1 "Cell polarity and asymmetric cell division: the *C. elegans* early embryo" by Anna Noatynska and Monica Gotta which considers how cell polarity is established in the model organism *C. elegans*. The next three chapters cover the mechanisms by which polarity in epithelial cells is regulated. Chapter 2 "Phosphoinositide lipids and cell polarity: linking the plasma membrane to the cytocortex" by Michael Krahn and Andreas Wodarz reviews the role of phospholipids in polarity. Chapter 3 "The role of secretory and endocytic pathways in the maintenance of cell polarity" by Su Fen Ang and Heike Fölsch and then our own Chapter 4 "Continuous endocytic recycling of tight junction proteins: how and why?" focus on the role of endocytic trafficking in maintaining epithelial polarity and junctions. The final chapter in this section, Chapter 5 "Crucial polarity regulators in axon specification" by Giovanna Lalli, provides an overview of polarity in axons, illustrating some interesting similarities between polarity in neurons and epithelial cells.

The second section starts with Chapter 6 "Cell wars: regulation of cell survival and proliferation by cell competition" by Silvia Vivarelli, Laura Wagstaff and Eugenia Piddini and provides a review of the fascinating process of cell competition in epithelial cells. The next two chapters, Chapter 7 "The control of gene expression and cell proliferation by the epithelial apical junctional complex" by Domenica Spadaro, Rocio Tapia, Pamela Pulimeno and Sandra Citi and Chapter 8 "Apicobasal polarity and cell proliferation during development" by Nitin Sabherwal and Nancy Papalopulu consider the important connections between epithelial polarity proteins and the regulation of proliferation. Chapter 9 "The Hippo pathway: key interaction and catalytic domains in organ growth control, stem cell self-renewal and tissue regeneration" by Claire Cherrett, Makoto Furutani-Seiki and Stefan Bagby focuses on the role of protein interactions and catalytic domains of Hippo signalling proteins, which play a key role in regulating epithelial growth. The volume finishes with two chapters, Chapter 10 "Epithelial cell polarity: what flies can teach us about cancer" by Daniel Bergstralh and Daniel St Johnston and Chapter 11 "The Scribble-Dlg-Lgl polarity module in development and cancer: from flies to man" by Imogen Elsum, Laura Yates, Patrick Humbert and Helena Richardson, which examine the links between polarity proteins and cancer formation. We feel that the 11 chapters provide a timely overview of this important field.

Many people helped to produce this volume and we thank the *Essays in Biochemistry* Editorial Advisory Panel and all members of the Portland Press staff. In particular Clare Curtis, who has been incredibly helpful and kept the whole process on track. We also thank the anonymous reviewers of the initial proposal and individual chapters and, of course, all of the authors for not just writing such high-quality reviews, but submitting them in a timely manner.

Andrew Chalmers and Paul Whitley
June 2012

Authors

Anna Noatynska is a postdoctoral fellow in Monica Gotta's laboratory (University of Geneva, Switzerland). She obtained her M.Sc. degree from Jagiellonian University (Krakow, Poland) and her Ph.D. from the University of Geneva (Switzerland). During her doctoral studies and her current postdoctoral work she has investigated the spatio-temporal co-ordination of cell-cycle progression and cell polarity during asymmetric cell division of the *C. elegans* early embryo. **Monica Gotta** did her undergraduate studies in Turin, Italy. She then moved to Switzerland where she investigated how nuclear organization influences gene expression. She received her Ph.D. from the University of Lausanne in 1997. She then joined the group of Dr Julie Ahringer at the Wellcome Trust/ Cancer Research UK Gurdon Institute to study the mechanisms of cell polarization and mitotic spindle positioning during asymmetric cell division of the *C. elegans* embryo. In 2002 she went back to Switzerland as a Swiss National Science Foundation Assistant Professor at the Institute of Biochemistry, ETH, Zurich. In 2008 she became Associate Professor at the Medical Faculty of the University of Geneva where she continues being fascinated by the process of asymmetric cell division.

Michael P. Krahn studied veterinary medicine at the Veterinary University (Tierärztliche Hochschule) of Hannover, Germany and obtained his Doctor of Veterinary Medicine in the laboratory of H.Y. Naim in 2006. He then moved to the University of Göttingen, Germany, where he obtained his Ph.D. in the laboratory of Andreas Wodarz in 2009. He continued to work in Göttingen, first as a postdoc and, from 2011, as junior group leader. In 2012 he was appointed Junior Professor of Anatomy and Cell Biology at the University of Regensburg, Germany. **Andreas Wodarz** studied Biology at the University of Cologne, Germany and obtained his Ph.D. in the laboratory of E. Knust in 1993. After his postdoc at Stanford University in the laboratory of R. Nusse he moved as a junior group leader to the University of Düsseldorf, Germany in 1997. Here he was appointed Assistant Professor of Genetics in 2001. In 2004 he accepted an offer to become Professor of Stem Cell Biology at the University of Göttingen, Germany. Since 2009 he has been Full Professor and Head of the Department of Anatomy and Cell Biology in Göttingen.

Su Fen Ang received her Ph.D. from the National University of Singapore and is currently a visiting postdoctoral fellow at the Feinberg School of Medicine, Northwestern University, Department of Cell and Molecular Biology. **Heike Fölsch** received her Ph.D. from the Ludwig–Maximilians University in Munich and is currently a Principal Investigator at the Feinberg School of Medicine, Northwestern University, Department of Cell and Molecular Biology.

Andrew D. Chalmers started his research career in 1996 as a Wellcome Prize Ph.D. student at the University of Bath where he investigated the development of the *Xenopus* digestive system. He then moved to a postdoctoral position at the Gurdon Institute, Cambridge and worked on epithelial polarity and asymmetric division. In 2004 he was awarded an MRC Career Development Fellowship and in 2005 an RCUK Academic Fellowship at the University of Bath. His group investigates the relationship between epithelial cell polarity, junctions and proliferation. This has involved a key collaboration with Dr Paul Whitley investigating the role of endosomal trafficking in polarity. **Paul Whitley** obtained his Ph.D. on protein secretion in yeast at the University of Edinburgh in 1991. He then took up postdoctoral positions at the Karolinska Institute (Novum) in Stockholm and Stockholm University working on membrane protein assembly. He moved to the Department of Clinical Immunology at the Karolinska Hospital/Institute before returning to the U.K. and the University of Bath in 1999. He has been a lecturer in the Department of Biology and Biochemistry at the University of Bath since 2000. His group is interested in endosomal trafficking and recently, in collaboration with Dr Andrew Chalmers, they have been investigating its role in cell polarity.

Giovanna Lalli obtained her Ph.D. in 2002 at Cancer Research UK, London, studying axonal retrograde transport in motor neurons. In 2003 she joined Alan Hall's group at the MRC Laboratory for Molecular and Cell Biology, University College London, where she investigated the role of the GTPase Ral in neurons. In 2007 she moved to King's College London, where she was awarded a King's College Young Investigator Fellowship. In 2010 she was appointed Lecturer in Molecular Neurobiology at King's College Wolfson Centre for Age-Related Diseases. Her research focuses on the molecular mechanisms regulating stem-cell-derived neural progenitor migration and differentiation.

Silvia Vivarelli graduated with an M.Sc. in Pharmaceutical Biotechnology from the University of Bologna (2005), and a Ph.D. in Translational and Molecular Medicine from the University of Milano (2010). Her M.Sc. thesis studies characterized two immobilized enzyme reactors inserted in an HPLC system, defining a high-throughput system to perform kinetic drug screenings. During her Ph.D. she characterized SRPK2, a kinase involved in pre-mRNA processing and the genotoxic stress cellular response. Since 2010 she has been working as a postdoc in Eugenia Piddini's laboratory. She is focusing on studying Wnt-mediated cell competition during tumorigenesis in mammalian cells.

Laura Wagstaff studied for her Ph.D. at the University of East Anglia (UEA) in Andrea Müsterberg's laboratory (2003–2006). Her research focused on the guidance signals for cardiac progenitor cells in early chick embryos. Two subsequent postdoctoral positions, also undertaken at UEA, promoted her interest in the field of cancer biology (Bass laboratory, 2006–2007, and Edwards laboratory, 2009–2010). Since June 2010 she has been a postdoc in Eugenia Piddini's laboratory (Gurdon Institute, Cambridge) studying the role of cell competition in Wnt-induced cancers. **Eugenia Piddini** was born and grew up in Sicily and studied cell and developmental biology at the University of Palermo. In 1997 she moved to Germany and did a Ph.D. in cell biology at the European Molecular Biology Laboratory in Heidelberg. She moved to London in 2002 and did her postdoctoral studies at the National Institute for Medical Research. There she worked on the regulation of tissue growth and patterning. Since 2010, she has been a Group Leader at the Gurdon Institute, University of Cambridge. Her laboratory investigates the molecular mechanisms of cell competition and its relevance to tissue biology.

Domenica Spadaro holds a Master's Degree in Biological Sciences from the University of Pavia, Italy, and is currently a Ph.D. student in the University of Geneva International Ph.D. Programme, in the group of Dr Sandra Citi. **Rocio Tapia** holds a B.S. Degree in Chemistry and Biology from the Universidad Benito Juarez de Oaxaca, and a Ph.D. in Molecular and Cellular Physiology from the CINVESTAV (Centro de Investigacion y de Estudios Avanzados del Istituto Politecnico Nacional), Mexico City (Mexico), and is currently a postdoctoral fellow in the group of Dr Sandra Citi. **Pamela Pulimeno** holds a Master's Degree in Biotechnology from the University of Genova, and a Ph.D. from the University of Geneva (Switzerland) in the group of Dr Sandra Citi, and is currently a postdoctoral fellow at the University of Geneva. **Sandra Citi** holds Biology and Medical Doctor degrees from the University of Florence (Italy), and a Ph.D. from the MRC Laboratory of Molecular Biology (Cambridge, U.K.). After a postdoctoral fellowship at the Weizmann Institute of Science, she has been a group leader, and held Senior Lecturer and Professor positions at Cornell University Medical College (New York, U.S.A.), the University of Padova (Italy) and the University of Geneva (Switzerland).

Nitin Sabherwal did his Ph.D. in the Institute of Human Genetics, University of Heidelberg, Germany, with Professor Gudrun Rappold, working on the regulation of short stature homeobox transcription factor (SHOX). After finishing his Ph.D. he joined the laboratory of Professor Nancy Papalopulu as a postdoctoral research associate. His main interest is apicobasal polarity signalling in embryonic and somatic cells during development and cancer. **Nancy Papalopulu** did her Ph.D. at the National Institute for Medical Research, U.K., with Dr Robb Krumlauf, on the role of homeobox genes in patterning the vertebrate central nervous system. She then joined the laboratory of Dr Chris Kintner at the Salk Institute for Biomedical Research, CA, U.S.A. with an HFSPO postdoctoral fellowship. In 1997 she became a group leader at the Wellcome Trust/Cancer Research UK Gurdon Institute in Cambridge, as a Wellcome Trust Career Development Fellow and subsequently, a Senior Research Fellow. Since 2006, she has been a Professor of Developmental Neuroscience at the University of Manchester. Her main interest is the molecular control of vertebrate neurogenesis.

Claire Cherrett (née Webb) has just completed her Ph.D. at the University of Bath, working with Stefan Bagby, Jean van den Elsen and Makoto Furutani-Seiki.

Claire worked on structure and function of Hippo pathway proteins using both NMR spectroscopy and X-ray crystallography. **Makoto Furutani-Seiki** has been at the University of Bath since 2007. He holds an MRC Senior Non-Clinical Fellowship. He previously did MD and Ph.D. degrees in Japan, post-doctoral work with Christiane Nüsslein-Volhard in Tübingen, and held group leader positions in Germany and Japan, where he was involved with large-scale mutagenesis screens in both zebrafish and medaka fish. His group uses medaka fish as a model organism to study the cellular and molecular mechanisms of organ growth control. **Stefan Bagby** has been at the University of Bath since 1999. Before that, he did a D.Phil. with Allen Hill in Oxford, followed by postdoctoral work with Mitsu Ikura in Toronto on structure and function of transcription factors and calcium-binding proteins. His group has been studying WW and C2 domains of Hippo pathway proteins.

Daniel Bergstralh began his research career as an NIH predoctoral fellow in Paul Roche's laboratory at the National Cancer Institute in Bethesda, MD, U.S.A. This was followed by doctoral work in cancer biology and immunology in Jenny Ting's laboratory at the University of North Carolina at Chapel Hill. He worked as a postdoc studying DNA repair with Jeff Sekelsky, also at UNC, and is currently in Daniel St Johnston's laboratory at the Gurdon Institute. He is also a Research Fellow at Clare Hall, University of Cambridge. **Daniel St Johnston** is the Director of the Wellcome Trust/Cancer Research UK Gurdon Institute at the University of Cambridge and a Wellcome Trust Principal Research Fellow. He obtained his Ph.D. from Harvard University in 1988, followed by a postdoc with Christiane Nüsslein Volhard studying *Drosophila* axis formation. He has been a group leader at the Gurdon Institute since 1991, where his group investigates how cells become polarized, how PAR proteins control the organization of the cytoskeleton and how mRNAs are targeted to the correct positions within the cell. He is a fellow of the Royal Society and member of EMBO.

Imogen Elsum is a postdoctoral researcher in Dr Patrick Humbert's laboratory at the Peter MacCallum Cancer Center, where she is carrying out research on the role of Scrib in tight junctions and the effect of Scrib loss-of-function in lung cancer. She received her Ph.D. with Dr Humbert in 2010 for her work concerning the mechanisms underlying the co-operation between Scrib and the oncogene Ras. **Laura Yates** is a postdoctoral researcher in Dr Patrick Humbert's laboratory at the Peter MacCallum Cancer Center, where she focuses on the relationship between PCP genes and Scrib in development and tumorigenesis. She carried out her Ph.D. in Dr Charlotte Dean's laboratory at MRC, Harwell, Oxfordshire, U.K., on the role of PCP regulators in mouse organ development. **Patrick Humbert** is a group leader at the Peter MacCallum Cancer Center, focusing on delineating the mechanism by which the Scribble polarity module regulates cellular signalling and cell polarity, using mammalian cell and mouse models. He received his Ph.D. at the Walter and Eliza Hall

Institute, Melbourne, and carried out postdoctoral research at the M.I.T. Center for Cancer Research, Cambridge, MA, U.S.A., in Dr Jacquie Lees's laboratory on cell-cycle regulation using mouse models. He set up his laboratory at the Peter MacCallum Cancer Center in 2000. **Helena Richardson** is a Group Leader at the Peter MacCallum Cancer Centre, where she uses the vinegar (fruit) fly, *Drosophila*, to model tumorigenesis, focusing on the Scribble polarity module. She received her Ph.D. at Adelaide University, South Australia, and carried out postdoctoral research with Dr Steve Reed at Scripps Research Institute, CA, U.S.A., on the control of cell proliferation in yeast and then with Dr Pat O'Farrell at University of California, San Francisco, CA, U.S.A., on cell proliferation in *Drosophila*. On returning to Adelaide, Australia, she worked in association with Dr Robert Saint on *Drosophila* cell proliferation and collaborated with Dr Sharad Kumar on *Drosophila* cell death regulation, before setting up her laboratory in Melbourne in 2000.

Abbreviations

ABCP	apico–basal cell polarity
ACD	asymmetric cell division
AEE	apical early endosome
AJ	adherens junction
AJC	apical junctional complex
AMOT	angiomotin
AMPK	AMP-activated kinase
AP	adaptor protein
APC	adenomatous polyposis coli
aPKC	atypical protein kinase C
Arf	ADP-ribosylation factor
ARH	autosomal recessive hypercholesterolaemia
A-VSVG	apical variant of the vesicular stomatitis virus glycoprotein
Baz	Bazooka
BEE	basolateral early endosome
BMP	bone morphogenetic protein
BP	basal progenitor
Cdc/CDC	cell division cycle
CDK	cyclin-dependent kinase
CDKI	cyclin-dependent kinase inhibitor
C-domain	central domain
CLIP	cytoplasmic linker protein
CNF-1	cytotoxic necrotizing factor-1
CP	cortical plate
Crb	Crumbs
CRMP2	collapsin-response-mediator protein 2
DAG	diacylglycerol
Dap160	dynamin-associated protein 160
DBD	DNA-binding domain
Dg	dystroglycan
Diap1	*Drosophila* inhibitor of apoptosis
DIC	differential interference contrast
Dlg	discs large
DOCK	dedicator of cytokinesis protein
dSPARC	*Drosophila* secreted protein acidic and rich in cysteine
Dvl/Dsh	Dishevelled
DYN	dynamin
ECM	extracellular matrix
ECT-2	epithelial cell transforming sequence 2

EE	early endosome
EGF	epidermal growth factor
EGFR	EGF receptor
EMT	epithelial–mesenchymal transition
E4-ORF1	*E4* region-encoded open reading frame 1
ERK	extracellular-signal-regulated kinase
ESCRT	endosomal sorting complex required for transport
Ex	Expanded
F-actin	filamentous actin
GAP	GTPase-activating protein
GEF	guanine-nucleotide-exchange factor
GIT1	G-protein-coupled receptor kinase-interacting Arf (ADP-ribosylation factor)-GAP (GTPase-activating protein) 1
GMC	ganglion mother cell
GPI	glycosylphosphatidylinositol
GPR	G-protein regulator
GSK	glycogen synthase kinase
GUK	guanylate kinase-like
HA	haemagglutinin
HSPC	haemopoietic stem and progenitor cell
HTLV-1	human T-cell leukaemia virus type 1
IFNγ	interferon γ
IFT	intraflagellar transport
IKNM	interkinetic nuclear migration
INPP5E	inositol polyphosphate-5-phosphatase E
IZ	intermediate zone
JAM	junctional adhesion molecule
JNK	c-Jun N-terminal kinase
KIF5	kinesin-5
LATS	large tumour suppressor
LDLR	LDL (low-density lipoprotein) receptor
Lef	lymphoid enhancer factor
LET	LEThal
LGL/Lgl	lethal giant larvae
LIN	abnormal cell LINeage
LKB1/Lkb1	liver kinase B1
LRR	leucine-rich repeat
MAGUK	membrane-associated guanylate kinase
MAP	microtubule-associated protein
MAPK	mitogen-activated protein kinase
MARK	MAP-regulating kinase
MDCK	Madin–Darby canine kidney
MEK	MAPK/ERK kinase

MEX	muscle excess
MOB1	Mps one binder
MSC	mesenchymal stem cell
MST	mammalian Ste (sterile) 20-like
Mud	Mushroom body defective
MUPP1	multi-PDZ-domain protein 1
NB	neuroblast
NgCAM	neuron glia cell adhesion molecule
Pak-1	p21-activated kinase-1
PALS1	protein associated with lin seven 1
PAR	PARtitioning defective
PCP	planar cell polarity
p120-ctn	p120-catenin
PDK1	phosphoinositide-dependent kinase 1
P-domain	peripheral area
PDZ	PSD-95 (postsynaptic density 95), Dlg (discs large) and ZO-1
PH	pleckstrin homology
Phlpp	PH (pleckstrin homology) domain and LRR protein phosphatase
PIKfyve	FYVE finger-containing phosphoinositide kinase
PI3K	phosphoinositide 3-kinase
PIE	pharynx and intestine excess
pIgR	polymeric Ig (immunoglobulin) receptor
PIPKIγ-90	PtdIns4P 5-kinase
PKA	protein kinase A
PKB	protein kinase B
PKC	protein kinase C
PLC	phospholipase C
PLK-1	Polo-Like Kinase 1
PNM	pronuclei meeting
PP2A	protein phosphatase 2A
PPARγ	peroxisome-proliferator-activated receptor γ
PTEN	phosphatase and tensin homologue deleted on chromosome 10
PTK7	protein tyrosine kinase 7
RE	recycling endosome
RNAi	RNA interference
ROCK	Rho-associated kinase
SAD	synapses of the amphid defective
Scrib/*scrib*	*scribble*
Sdt	Stardust
SH3	Src homology 3
Sqh	spaghetti-squash
Sra 1	specifically Rac1-associated protein 1

SRF	serum response factor
STEF	Sif and Tiam1-like exchange factor
SVZ	subventricular zone
TAD	transcription activation domain
TAZ	transcriptional coactivator with PDZ-binding motif
TBD	TEAD-binding domain
TCF	T-cell factor
T2DM	Type 2 diabetes mellitus
TfnR	Tfn (transferrin) receptor
TGFβ	transforming growth factor β
TGN	*trans*-Golgi network
+TIP	plus-end tracking protein
TJ	tight junction
T-zone	transition zone
UBA	ubiquitin-associated
VZ	ventricular zone
WAVE	WASP (Wiskott–Aldrich syndrome protein) verprolin homologous
YAP	Yes-associated protein
YBD	YAP-binding domain
ZA	zonula adherens
ZO	zonula occludens
ZONAB	ZO-1-associated nucleic acid-binding protein

© The Authors Journal compilation © 2012 Biochemical Society
Essays Biochem. (2012) **53**, 1–14: doi: 10.1042/BSE0530001

Cell polarity and asymmetric cell division: the *C. elegans* early embryo

Anna Noatynska and Monica Gotta[1]

Department of Physiology and Metabolism, Faculty of Medicine, University of Geneva, 1 rue Michel Servet, 1211 Geneva 4, Switzerland

Abstract

Cell polarity is crucial for many functions including cell migration, tissue organ-ization and asymmetric cell division. In animal cells, cell polarity is controlled by the highly conserved PAR (PARtitioning defective) proteins. *par* genes have been identified in *Caenorhabditis elegans* in screens for maternal lethal muta-tions that disrupt cytoplasmic partitioning and asymmetric division. Although PAR proteins were identified more than 20 years ago, our understanding on how they regulate polarity and how they are regulated is still incomplete. In this chapter we review our knowledge of the processes of cell polarity establishment and maintenance, and asymmetric cell division in the early *C. elegans* embryo. We discuss recent findings that highlight new players in cell polarity and/or reveal the molecular details on how PAR proteins regulate polarity processes.

Introduction

Cell polarization is achieved by an unequal distribution of cellular factors (mRNA, proteins) and/or organelles along a cellular axis. Signals inducing

[1]To whom correspondence should be addressed (email monica.gotta@unige.ch).

cell polarization (intrinsic, e.g. [1,2] or extrinsic, e.g. [3]) create distinct cellular domains which in turn determine the leading edge during migration, confer the directionality of transport and/or secretion of molecules within the tissue, or ensure the distribution of cell-fate determinants. Thus cell polarity is essential for the function of almost all cell types and, when perturbed, can lead to disease [4,5].

Cell polarization is also one of the prerequisites for asymmetric (unequal) cell division, a crucial biological process required to generate diversity during development. A cell divides asymmetrically when it gives rise to daughter cells with distinct developmental potentials. Examples of asymmetric cell division can be found within diverse species including bacteria (e.g. *Caulobacter crescentus* division [6]), unicellular eukaryotic organisms (e.g. *Saccharomyces cerevisiae* division [7]) and invertebrates (e.g. *Caenorhabditis elegans* and *Drosophila melanogaster* [8]), as well as in plants and algae (e.g. *Arabidopsis thaliana* and *Fucus serratus* [9]), and finally mammals [10].

The majority of unequal divisions create cells different in size. Most importantly, however, daughter cells inherit distinct cell-fate determinants that drive their diverse developmental programmes. The two main requirements for a successful asymmetric cell division are: (i) cell polarization along a predetermined axis and (ii) orientation of the mitotic spindle along the polarity axis (Figure 1).

The molecular mechanisms governing polarity and asymmetric cell division, although highly conserved and extensively investigated in different systems, are not yet completely understood. Studies on model organisms have contributed enormously to our understanding of the polarity network, which controls cell fate across species [8]. In the present chapter we review the mechanisms regulating cell polarity establishment and maintenance, and asymmetric cell division in the *C. elegans* one-cell embryo.

Early development of the *C. elegans* embryo

The *C. elegans* early embryo is an excellent model to investigate the molecular mechanisms governing polarity and asymmetric cell division. The first embryonic division is asymmetric and completed approximately 30 min after fertilization. In addition, embryonic divisions are highly stereotypical and can be followed in real time using Nomarski optics [DIC (differential interference contrast); Figures 1A–1G].

The development of the embryo starts when the oocyte, arrested in prophase of meiosis I, is fertilized while passing through the spermatheca. Upon fertilization, both meiotic divisions are completed and two polar bodies are extruded from the zygote. The sperm, which provides the centrosomes to the embryo, fertilize the oocyte usually on the opposite side to the oocyte nucleus. Centrosomes and associated microtubules define the future posterior pole of the embryo and therefore the first axis of polarity, the anterior–posterior axis. Following sperm entry, the acto-myosin cytoskeleton undergoes rapid rearrangements, which result in strong ruffling of the cortex (Figures 1A, 1B,

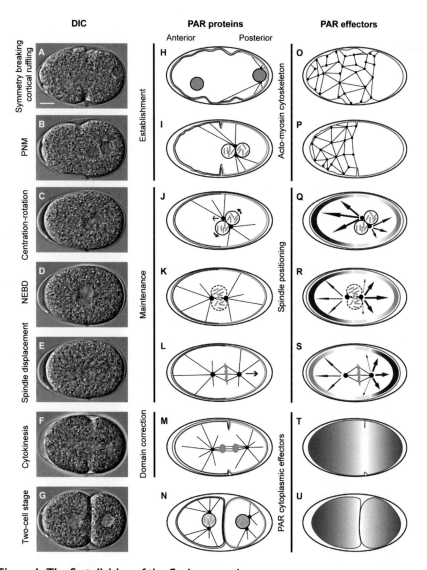

Figure 1. The first division of the *C. elegans* embryo

(**A–G**) Still images from a DIC movie of a wild-type *C. elegans* embryo. The worm embryo is surrounded by an impermeable eggshell. Embryos are approximately 50 μm long, transparent and undergo rapid development. The developmental stage is indicated on the left-hand side. (**H–N**) Corresponding schematic drawings of the DIC stages with the addition of cortical PAR proteins: anterior (PAR-3–PAR-6–PKC-3) in red and posterior (PAR-1–PAR-2) in green. (**O** and **P**) Myosin dynamics, (**Q–S**) pronuclei centration, rotation and spindle positioning, (**T** and **U**) cytoplasmic factors. Black dots in (**H–N**) and (**Q–S**) represent centrosomes, the black lines represent associated microtubules and DNA is light blue; (**O** and **P**) acto-myosin network; (**Q–S**) dynamic localization of GPR-1/2, LIN-5 (dark blue) and LET-99 (yellow); (**T** and **U**) cell-fate determinants enriched in the anterior (violet) and posterior (pink) cytoplasm in the one-cell embryo (**T**) and subsequently in AB and P1 (**U**). Arrows indicate: rotation and movement of the pronuclei and centrosomes (**J**); posterior displacement of the mitotic spindle (**L**); and pulling forces exerted on spindle poles (**Q–S**). Note that in (**Q–S**), the thickness of the arrows is proportional to the intensity of forces. Anterior is on the left, posterior is on the right. Scale bar = 10 μm. NEBD, nuclear envelope breakdown.

1O and 1P). Meanwhile, the maternal and paternal pronuclei grow in size and become clearly noticeable by DIC (Figure 1A). While the ruffling of the cortex culminates in one pronounced invagination in the middle of the embryo (pseudocleavage), the female pronucleus starts migrating towards the posterior pole to meet the sperm pronucleus. The two pronuclei meet in the posterior half of the embryo [PNM (pronuclei meeting); Figure 1B] and migrate together towards the centre of the embryo while rotating 90° to align the centrosomes along the polarity axis (Figures 1C and 1J). Subsequently, nuclear envelopes break down (Figures 1D and 1K), the mitotic spindle sets up, elongates and is pulled to the posterior, while the posterior spindle pole exhibits oscillations along the short axis of the embryo (Figures 1E and 1L). Finally, the cytokinetic furrow ingresses in the posterior part of the embryo (Figure 1F), bisecting the spindle and creating two cells with unequal size, a bigger anterior (AB) and a smaller posterior (P1) cell (Figure 1G).

AB and P1 inherit distinct factors that specify different developmental fates (Figure 1N and see below). The anterior cell will divide symmetrically and give rise to somatic tissues. Conversely, the posterior cell will continue to divide asymmetrically to finally create two germ cell precursors and somatic cells. AB and P1 also differ in cell-cycle timing and spindle orientation. The AB cell divides approximately 2 min before P1 cells, and the mitotic spindle of AB cells is perpendicular, whereas the spindle of the P1 cell is parallel, to the polarity axis [11]. All of these processes are under the control of the highly conserved PAR (PARtitioning defective) proteins [12].

PAR proteins: major polarity players

PAR proteins are major players orchestrating cell polarity and asymmetric division. They were identified in *C. elegans* in genetic screens for regulators of asymmetric division of the one-cell zygote. The *par* mutants are unable to establish and/or maintain polarity, they display developmental defects and eventually die [13]. Until now seven master polarity proteins have been identified: PAR-1 to PAR-6 and PKC-3 (atypical protein kinase C, also known as aPKC). Subsequent studies in other organisms identified homologues of PAR proteins (with the exception of PAR-2), suggesting that they are part of a universal machinery governing cellular polarity (reviewed in [12]).

In *C. elegans* early embryos five PAR proteins are asymmetrically distributed forming physically and functionally distinct domains (Figures 1H–1N and 2). The anterior cortex is occupied by the dynamic complex of PKC-3 [14], and two PDZ-domain containing proteins, PAR-3 and PAR-6 (Figures 1H–1M and 2) [15–17]. The posterior pole is occupied by PAR-1, a serine/threonine protein kinase [18], and PAR-2, a RING finger protein (Figures 1H–1M and 2) [19–21]. The serine/threonine kinase PAR-4 and a member of the 14-3-3 family, PAR-5, are uniformly distributed through the cortex and in the cytoplasm [22,23]. The localization of PAR proteins in the one-cell embryo proceeds in two temporally and mechanistically distinct stages: the establishment and the maintenance phase (Figure 1) [24], as described below.

Polarity establishment

In newly fertilized embryos the PAR-3–PAR-6–PKC-3 complex is found all around the cortex, and PAR-1 and PAR-2 are in the cytoplasm [21,24]. A net of symmetrically distributed acto-myosin foci decorates the cortex of the entire embryo and drives cortical contractions and ruffling [11,25]. Cortical contractions depend on the activity of the small G-protein RHO-1, regulated by the GEF (guanine-nucleotide-exchange factor) ECT-2 (epithelial cell transforming sequence 2), and the GAPs (GTPase-activating proteins) RGA-3 and RGA-4 (RGA is Rho GAP), all of which are localized at the cortex [26–30].

Polarity establishment is initiated by the paternally provided centrosome, which brings the signal to break the cortical and cytoplasmic symmetries. The molecular nature of this signal is not clear [31,32]. Nevertheless, the sperm-donated centrosome and associated microtubules contact the posterior cortex and trigger the local inhibition of cortical contractions [21,27,33–37], which results in a progressive relaxation of the posterior cortex and displacement of contractile centres towards the anterior pole, a process referred to as cytoplasmic flows (Figures 1A, 1B, 1O and 1P) [24,38,39]. The flows transport PAR-3–PAR-6–PKC-3 to the anterior and enable PAR-2, and subsequently PAR-1, to associate with the posterior cortex (Figures 1H and 1I) [24,38,40].

PAR proteins are important for polarity establishment. The anterior PAR proteins play a major role as polarity fails to be established in *par-3*, *par-6* or *pkc-3* mutants. Anterior PAR proteins also amplify cortical flows, further promoting their own transport towards the anterior pole [38,40]. In wild-type PAR-2 microtubule binding helps its own recruitment to the cortex nearest to the centrosomes, contributing to efficient polarity establishment [21]. In the absence of ECT-2-dependent cortical flows, PAR-2 becomes essential to break embryonic symmetries [21,41]. PAR-4 positively regulates the acto-myosin contractility and thus contributes to polarity establishment (Figure 2) [42]. Finally, PAR-5 also participates in the establishment phase as, in *par-5*-depleted embryos, the PAR-3 complex clears the posterior less efficiently [23,24].

An unanswered question is how PAR proteins interact with the cortex. *C. elegans* embryos lacking PAR-6 or PKC-3 display a residual cortical presence of PAR-3, whereas depletion of PAR-3 completely abolishes the peripheral localization of PAR-6 and PKC-3 [14,15]. PAR-3 could therefore serve as a scaffold protein. Studies in human cells and in *Drosophila* showed that PAR-3 can bind phospholipids *in vitro* [43,44] and has the ability to oligomerize [17,45,46]. Thus PAR-3 could be loaded on the cortex by interacting with phospholipids and subsequently recruit PAR-6 and PKC-3. At the posterior, PAR-2 loads on the cortex (possibly by phospholipid binding) and subsequently localizes PAR-1 [21].

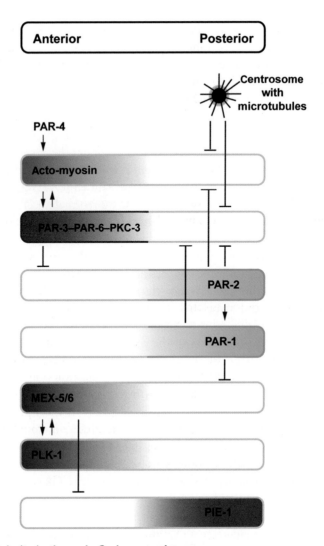

Figure 2. Polarity in the early *C. elegans* embryo
Regulatory relationships between PAR proteins and their downstream targets which drive asymmetric division in the early *C. elegans* embryo. Anterior and posterior PAR proteins exert inhibitory interactions on each other. The cortical PAR asymmetry governs the localization of several cytoplasmic proteins. Lines with bars, inhibitory interactions; arrows, postitive regulation; darker and lighter colours illustrate higher and lower levels of the protein respectively (based on data from [24]). Not shown: (i) LGL-1, a non-essential gene which works redundantly with PAR-2 [53,54]; and (ii) PAR-5 in establishment and maintenance of polarity [24] and the feedback regulation between PAR proteins and MEX-5/6 [61,63] or PLK-1 [75].

Establishment of polarity and PAR cortical binding are also regulated by the Hsp90 (heat-shock protein 90) co-chaperone CDC-37 (Cdc is cell division cycle) [47]. In embryos depleted of *cdc-37* by RNAi (RNA interference) [*cdc-37(RNAi)*], PAR-3 initially clears up from the posterior, but PAR-6 and PKC-3 remain high around the cortex, indicating that CDC-37 is required for proper interaction between the anterior PAR proteins [47].

Thus cortical flows localize PAR-3, PAR-6 and PKC-3 to the anterior cortical half of the embryo. Concomitantly, PAR-2 and PAR-1 associate with the posterior cortex. At the end of the establishment phase (around the PNM stage), the anterior–posterior PAR domains are well defined, non-overlapping and each of them occupy approximately 50% of the embryonic cortex (Figure 1I) [24].

Polarity maintenance

Although segregated to the anterior and posterior (Figure 1I), PAR proteins are not stably bound to the cortex, they can diffuse laterally and rapidly exchange with the cytoplasmic pool [40,48]. Polarity is maintained by a complex network of interactions, which counterbalances the dynamic behaviour of PAR proteins.

PAR-2 plays a major role in the maintenance phase. To prevent the invasion of the anterior complex towards the posterior, PAR-2 (i) inhibits the re-assembly of acto-myosin foci in the posterior pole, which, if it occurred, would trigger abnormal posterior-directed flows and the re-distribution of PAR-3–PAR-6–PKC-3 to the posterior cortex [38] and (ii) localizes to the posterior cortex PAR-1, which phosphorylates PAR-3 and thus contributes to exclude the anterior complex from the PAR-1–PAR-2 domain [21]. In turn, PKC-3 phosphorylates PAR-2 and inhibits its anterior localization (Figure 2) [49].

PAR-5 is also involved in polarity maintenance, although its molecular targets are not known. It is plausible, however, that PAR-5 binds phosphorylated PAR-1 to exclude it from the anterior or PAR-3 to exclude it from the posterior, similar to *Drosophila* and mammalian cells [50–52].

LGL-1, the homologue of *Drosophila lgl* (Lethal Giant Larvae), also participates in maintenance of polarity [53,54]. Although LGL-1 is not essential for embryonic development, its depletion increases the embryonic lethality and the polarity defects of a weak *par-2* mutant, whereas its overexpression rescues PAR-2 depletion by restoring embryonic polarity [53,54]. LGL-1 co-immunoprecipitates with PAR-6 and PKC-3; however, it localizes to the opposite posterior cortex [53,54]. The model suggests that LGL-1 forms a complex with PKC-3 and PAR-6 at the boundary between PAR domains. This allows phosphorylation of LGL-1 by PKC-3 and makes the LGL-1–PKC-3–PAR-6 complex dissociate from the cortex, inhibiting spreading of the anterior complex to the posterior LGL-1–PAR-2 domain [54]. In addition, similarly to PAR-2, LGL-1 contributes to inhibit the re-assembly of acto-myosin foci in the posterior of the embryo, and thus prevents posteriorly directed flows and re-distribution of the anterior complex to the posterior pole after the PNM stage [53,54].

CDC-37 is also involved in polarity maintenance as reducing its levels impairs the mutual exclusion between anterior and posterior complexes. As CDC-37-depleted embryos show lower PKC-3 levels, it is possible that, in *cdc-37(RNAi)* embryos, PAR-2 is less efficiently phosphorylated by PKC-3 and thus cannot be excluded from the anterior cortex ([47] and see below).

Polarity maintenance also depends on the small GTPase CDC-42 [26,55,56]. CDC-42 binds to PAR-6 and promotes its localization at the cortex, stabilizing the anterior complex during the maintenance phase [55–57].

Finally, spatio–temporal regulation of endocytosis is also crucial to maintain membrane asymmetries. DYN-1 (the orthologue of dynamin, a large GTPase [58]) regulates endocytosis and is enriched in the anterior cortex in one-cell embryos [59]. In DYN-1-depleted embryos, the anteriorly enriched endocytic events, present in wild-type, are altered and polarity is lost. DYN-1 may regulate internalization and recycling of PAR-6, therefore restricting it to the anterior domain [59].

At the end of the maintenance phase, the cytokinetic furrow ingresses in the posterior half of the embryo (Figures 1F and 1M). To properly segregate cell-fate determinants into daughter cells, cell polarity must be coupled with the site of cytokinetic furrow ingression. To achieve this co-ordination, PAR proteins control the position of the mitotic spindle (see below). As an additional mechanism, the cytokinetic furrow senses the PAR-2 boundary and is able to correct its position (Figure 1M) [60]. This mechanism depends on heterotrimeric G-proteins (see below) and ensures that the cytokinetic furrow matches the border between the posterior and the anterior PAR domains, asymmetrically separating them into the sister cells: the PAR-3–PAR-6–PKC-3 to the AB cell and PAR-2–PAR-1 to the P1 cell (Figure 1N) [24,60].

In summary, phosphorylation-dependent mutual inhibition of the anterior and posterior PAR proteins, regulation of endocytosis and myosin assembly/disassembly all contribute to maintain polarity in the one-cell embryo.

PAR protein downstream effectors

PAR protein asymmetry governs unequal segregation of several cytoplasmic proteins (including cell-fate determinants; Figure 1T) and thus guarantees their proper distribution into the daughter cells [11]. Two CCCH zinc-finger proteins MEX-5 (MEX is Muscle Excess) and MEX-6 (highly similar in protein sequence and function hereafter referred as MEX-5/6) [61] and the mitotic kinase PLK-1 (Polo-Like Kinase 1) [62–65] form an anterior-to-posterior gradient in the one-cell embryo and are segregated to the AB cell. By contrast, other CCCH zinc-finger proteins form a posterior-to-anterior gradient and are subsequently segregated into the P1 cell [66,67]. A fundamental question is how cytoplasmic gradients are generated and maintained.

Previous studies show that a difference in diffusion rate can establish and maintain such gradients [68–71]. In the one-cell embryo, the diffusion coefficient of PIE-1 (PIE is Pharynx and Intestine Excess), a CCCH protein that represses transcription [72,73], is lower in the posterior than in the anterior, resulting in a posterior-to-anterior gradient. The authors postulate that the lower diffusion coefficient may be a consequence of PIE-1 binding to RNAs in the posterior cytoplasm [69].

The MEX-5 anterior-to-posterior gradient also depends on diffusivity [68,70,71], which is controlled by the PAR-1 kinase [68,70,71] and uniformly distributed PP2A (Protein Phosphatase 2A) [71]. In the posterior, MEX-5 phosphorylated by PAR-1 is released from slow-diffusive RNA-containing complexes and thus exhibits faster mobility. In the anterior, however, PAR-1 is absent and MEX-5, dephosphorylated by PP2A, can associate with slow-diffusive complexes. Therefore, owing to the antagonistic action of PAR-1 and PP2A, MEX-5 diffuses faster from the posterior to the anterior pole than in the opposite direction, generating a concentration gradient [71].

The asymmetric localization of these proteins is crucial for embryonic patterning. For instance, PIE-1 is restricted to the germline lineage where it represses transcription [72,73]. MEX-5 binds to PLK-1 and promotes its localization to the anterior pole, and thus the AB cell [63]. The enrichment of PLK-1 in AB is crucial for the asynchronous mitotic entry of AB and P1 [64,65], which in turn is important for the respective positioning and cell–cell contacts of descendant daughter cells [74]. A feedback regulation between PAR proteins, MEX-5 and downstream effectors also exists. MEX-5 promotes the growth of the PAR-2 domain during polarity establishment [24], whereas PLK-1 activates MEX-5 [63] and influences localization of PAR proteins [63,75]. Such a complex network of interactions is crucial for *C. elegans* development, and once perturbed leads to defective differentiation and death.

Positioning of the mitotic spindle and unequal cell division

The first division of the *C. elegans* zygote creates cells different in content and in size. To do so, the mitotic spindle of the one-cell embryo is firstly orientated along the polarity axis and subsequently pulled towards the posterior pole to dictate asymmetric cleavage and thus unequally segregate polarized factors (Figures 1E and 1L) [76]. Interactions between the cortex and astral microtubules are important for both events. Forces generated at the cortex, which pull on astral microtubules, involve a set of conserved proteins: dynein (a microtubule minus-end motor), GOA-1 (GOA is G-Protein O, α subunit) and GPA-16 (GPA is G-Protein α subunit) (two redundant G_α proteins), GPR-1 and GPR-2 (GPR is G-Protein Regulator) (two almost identical G_α regulators, hereafter referred as GPR-1/2) and LIN-5 (LIN is abnormal cell LINeage) (a coiled-coil protein) (reviewed in [8,77]).

Although G_α subunits are symmetrically distributed, its activators display dynamic and cell-cycle-dependent localization (Figures 1Q–1S). Until metaphase GPR-1/2 and LIN-5 are enriched at the anterior cortex to align centrosomes with the anterior–posterior axis (Figure 1Q) [78–80], whereas, in metaphase and anaphase, GPR-1/2 and LIN-5 become enriched at the posterior and drive posterior spindle displacement (Figures 1R and 1S [79], reviewed in [77]). PKC-3 phosphorylates LIN-5 and thus inhibits cortical pulling forces in the anterior pole [81]. In addition, pulling forces are diminished on the lateral–posterior cortex by LET-99 (LEThal 99) a DEP (Dishevelled, Egl-10 and Pleckstrin) domain protein, which negatively regulates the localization of GPR-1/2, therefore inhibiting lateral pulling on astral microtubules which is counterproductive for spindle positioning (Figures 1Q–1S, reviewed in [77]). In *par* mutants the asymmetric localization of LIN-5 and GPR-1/2 is lost and the spindle remains in the centre of the cell, resulting in a symmetric first cleavage [82]. Therefore PAR proteins regulate asymmetric spindle positioning by controlling the localization and activity of LIN-5 and GPR-1/2.

Conclusions

PAR proteins regulate the process of asymmetric cell division. This does not only involve the establishment and the maintenance of cortical polarity, but also entails the proper distribution of downstream cell-fate determinants, alignment of the mitotic spindle with the axis of polarity, and co-ordination between cellular processes and cell-cycle progression. To do so, the cortical polarity of PAR proteins is transduced into the asymmetric distribution and/or activity of proteins controlling cell-cycle progression and cell fate.

PAR proteins act with partners and effectors to efficiently polarize cells. Identifying new partners and/or PAR effectors and addressing the co-ordination between PAR polarity and other processes during asymmetric cell division will lead us towards a better understanding of this process. Given that many proteins are highly conserved, it is plausible that similar mechanisms operate during mammalian development and asymmetric division of stem cells.

Summary

- *Cell polarity and asymmetric cell division are crucial to generate diversity during development.*
- *Successful asymmetric cell division requires establishment of a polarity axis, subsequent distribution of cell-fate determinants and orientation of the mitotic spindle along the axis of polarity.*
- *PAR proteins are major regulators orchestrating cell polarization, spindle orientation and asymmetric cell division across species. In the one-cell embryo PAR proteins form two reciprocal and mutually exclusive domains [anterior (PAR-3–PAR-6–PKC-3) and posterior (PAR-2–PAR-1)].*
- *Our understanding of cell polarity and asymmetric division is still incomplete. Identifying new interactors of PAR proteins and studying how, for instance, spindle orientation, cytokinesis, polarity establishment and maintenance are co-ordinated in space and time will lead us towards a better understanding of differentiation and stem cell biology, as well as disease development.*

We thank Lesilee Rose, Elsa Kress and Manoel Prouteau for critical reading of the chapter and many useful comments. We also thank the reviewers for their constructive criticisms. Research in the M.G. laboratory is supported by the Swiss National Science Foundation, by an EMBO YIP (Young Investigator Programme) grant and from the University of Geneva.

References

1. Slaughter, B.D., Smith, S.E. and Li, R. (2009) Symmetry breaking in the life cycle of the budding yeast. Cold Spring Harbor Perspect. Biol. **1**, a003384

2. Gulli, M.P. and Peter, M. (2001) Temporal and spatial regulation of Rho-type guanine-nucleotide exchange factors: the yeast perspective. Genes Dev. **15**, 365–379

3. Siegrist, S.E. and Doe, C.Q. (2006) Extrinsic cues orient the cell division axis in *Drosophila* embryonic neuroblasts. Development **133**, 529–536

4. Wilson, P.D. (2011) Apico-basal polarity in polycystic kidney disease epithelia. Biochim. Biophys. Acta **1812**, 1239–1248

5. Florian, M.C. and Geiger, H. (2010) Concise review: polarity in stem cells, disease, and aging. Stem Cells **28**, 1623–1629

6. Thanbichler, M. (2009). Spatial regulation in *Caulobacter crescentus*. Curr. Opin. Microbiol. **12**, 715–721

7. Barral, Y. and Liakopoulos, D. (2009) Role of spindle asymmetry in cellular dynamics. Int. Rev. Cell Mol. Biol. **278**, 149–213

8. Gonczy, P. (2008). Mechanisms of asymmetric cell division: flies and worms pave the way. Nat. Rev. **9**, 355–366

9. De Smet, I. and Beeckman, T. (2011) Asymmetric cell division in land plants and algae: the driving force for differentiation. Nat. Rev. **12**, 177–188

10. Neumuller, R.A. and Knoblich, J.A. (2009) Dividing cellular asymmetry: asymmetric cell division and its implications for stem cells and cancer. Genes Dev. **23**, 2675–2699

11. Gonczy, P. and Rose, L.S. (2005) Asymmetric cell division and axis formation in the embryo. WormBook, 1–20

12. Goldstein, B. and Macara, I.G. (2007) The PAR proteins: fundamental players in animal cell polarization. Dev. Cell **13**, 609–622

13. Kemphues, K.J., Priess, J.R., Morton, D.G. and Cheng, N.S. (1988). Identification of genes required for cytoplasmic localization in early *C. elegans* embryos. Cell **52**, 311–320

14. Tabuse, Y., Izumi, Y., Piano, F., Kemphues, K.J., Miwa, J. and Ohno, S. (1998) Atypical protein kinase C cooperates with PAR-3 to establish embryonic polarity in *Caenorhabditis elegans*. Development **125**, 3607–3614

15. Hung, T.J. and Kemphues, K.J. (1999) PAR-6 is a conserved PDZ domain-containing protein that colocalizes with PAR-3 in *Caenorhabditis elegans* embryos. Development **126**, 127–135

16. Etemad-Moghadam, B., Guo, S. and Kemphues, K.J. (1995) Asymmetrically distributed PAR-3 protein contributes to cell polarity and spindle alignment in early *C. elegans* embryos. Cell **83**, 743–752

17. Li, J., Kim, H., Aceto, D.G., Hung, J., Aono, S. and Kemphues, K.J. (2010) Binding to PKC-3, but not to PAR-3 or to a conventional PDZ domain ligand, is required for PAR-6 function in *C. elegans*. Dev. Biol. **340**, 88–98

18. Guo, S. and Kemphues, K.J. (1995) par-1, a gene required for establishing polarity in *C. elegans* embryos, encodes a putative Ser/Thr kinase that is asymmetrically distributed. Cell **81**, 611–620

19. Levitan, D.J., Boyd, L., Mello, C.C., Kemphues, K.J. and Stinchcomb, D.T. (1994) par-2, a gene required for blastomere asymmetry in *Caenorhabditis elegans*, encodes zinc-finger and ATP-binding motifs. Proc. Natl. Acad. Sci. U.S.A. **91**, 6108–6112

20. Boyd, L., Guo, S., Levitan, D., Stinchcomb, D.T. and Kemphues, K.J. (1996) PAR-2 is asymmetrically distributed and promotes association of P granules and PAR-1 with the cortex in *C. elegans* embryos. Development **122**, 3075–3084

21. Motegi, F., Zonies, S., Hao, Y., Cuenca, A.A., Griffin, E. and Seydoux, G. (2011) Microtubules induce self-organization of polarized PAR domains in *Caenorhabditis elegans* zygotes. Nat. Cell Biol. **13**, 1361–1367

22. Watts, J.L., Morton, D.G., Bestman, J. and Kemphues, K.J. (2000) The *C. elegans* par-4 gene encodes a putative serine-threonine kinase required for establishing embryonic asymmetry. Development **127**, 1467–1475

23. Morton, D.G., Shakes, D.C., Nugent, S., Dichoso, D., Wang, W., Golden, A. and Kemphues, K.J. (2002) The *Caenorhabditis elegans* par-5 gene encodes a 14-3-3 protein required for cellular asymmetry in the early embryo. Dev. Biol. **241**, 47–58

24. Cuenca, A.A., Schetter, A., Aceto, D., Kemphues, K. and Seydoux, G. (2003) Polarization of the *C. elegans* zygote proceeds via distinct establishment and maintenance phases. Development **130**, 1255–1265

25. Cowan, C.R. and Hyman, A.A. (2007) Acto-myosin reorganization and PAR polarity in *C. elegans*. Development **134**, 1035–1043

26. Motegi, F. and Sugimoto, A. (2006) Sequential functioning of the ECT-2 RhoGEF, RHO-1 and CDC-42 establishes cell polarity in *Caenorhabditis elegans* embryos. Nat. Cell Biol. **8**, 978–985

27. Jenkins, N., Saam, J.R. and Mango, S.E. (2006) CYK-4/GAP provides a localized cue to initiate anteroposterior polarity upon fertilization. Science **313**, 1298–1301

28. Schonegg, S. and Hyman, A.A. (2006) CDC-42 and RHO-1 coordinate acto-myosin contractility and PAR protein localization during polarity establishment in *C. elegans* embryos. Development **133**, 3507–3516

29. Schonegg, S., Constantinescu, A.T., Hoege, C. and Hyman, A.A. (2007) The Rho GTPase-activating proteins RGA-3 and RGA-4 are required to set the initial size of PAR domains in *Caenorhabditis elegans* one-cell embryos. Proc. Natl. Acad. Sci. U.S.A. **104**, 14976–14981

30. Schmutz, C., Stevens, J. and Spang, A. (2007). Functions of the novel RhoGAP proteins RGA-3 and RGA-4 in the germ line and in the early embryo of *C. elegans*. Development **134**, 3495–3505

31. Marston, D.J. and Goldstein, B. (2006) Symmetry breaking in *C. elegans*: another gift from the sperm. Dev. Cell **11**, 273–274

32. Munro, E. and Bowerman, B. (2009) Cellular symmetry breaking during *Caenorhabditis elegans* development. Cold Spring Harbor Perspect. Biol. **1**, a003400

33. O'Connell, K.F., Maxwell, K.N. and White, J.G. (2000) The spd-2 gene is required for polarization of the anteroposterior axis and formation of the sperm asters in the *Caenorhabditis elegans* zygote. Dev. Biol. **222**, 55–70

34. Wallenfang, M.R. and Seydoux, G. (2000) Polarization of the anterior-posterior axis of *C. elegans* is a microtubule-directed process. Nature **408**, 89–92

35. Tsai, M.C. and Ahringer, J. (2007) Microtubules are involved in anterior-posterior axis formation in *C. elegans* embryos. J. Cell Biol. **179**, 397–402

36. Cowan, C.R. and Hyman, A.A. (2004) Centrosomes direct cell polarity independently of microtubule assembly in *C. elegans* embryos. Nature **431**, 92–96

37. Fortin, S.M., Marshall, S.L., Jaeger, E.C., Greene, P.E., Brady, L.K., Isaac, R.E., Schrandt, J.C., Brooks, D.R. and Lyczak, R. (2010) The PAM-1 aminopeptidase regulates centrosome positioning to ensure anterior-posterior axis specification in one-cell *C. elegans* embryos. Dev. Biol. **344**, 992–1000

38. Munro, E., Nance, J. and Priess, J.R. (2004) Cortical flows powered by asymmetrical contraction transport PAR proteins to establish and maintain anterior-posterior polarity in the early *C. elegans* embryo. Dev. Cell **7**, 413–424

39. Xiong, H., Mohler, W.A. and Soto, M.C. (2011) The branched actin nucleator Arp2/3 promotes nuclear migrations and cell polarity in the *C. elegans* zygote. Dev. Biol. **357**, 356–369

40. Cheeks, R.J., Canman, J.C., Gabriel, W.N., Meyer, N., Strome, S. and Goldstein, B. (2004) *C. elegans* PAR proteins function by mobilizing and stabilizing asymmetrically localized protein complexes. Curr. Biol. **14**, 851–862

41. Zonies, S., Motegi, F., Hao, Y. and Seydoux, G. (2010) Symmetry breaking and polarization of the *C. elegans* zygote by the polarity protein PAR-2. Development **137**, 1669–1677

42. Chartier, N.T., Salazar Ospina, D.P., Benkemoun, L., Mayer, M., Grill, S.W., Maddox, A.S. and Labbe, J.C. (2011) PAR-4/LKB1 mobilizes nonmuscle myosin through anillin to regulate *C. elegans* embryonic polarization and cytokinesis. Curr. Biol. **21**, 259–269

43. Wu, H., Feng, W., Chen, J., Chan, L.N., Huang, S. and Zhang, M. (2007) PDZ domains of Par-3 as potential phosphoinositide signaling integrators. Mol. Cell **28**, 886–898

44. Krahn, M.P., Klopfenstein, D.R., Fischer, N. and Wodarz, A. (2010) Membrane targeting of Bazooka/PAR-3 is mediated by direct binding to phosphoinositide lipids. Curr. Biol. **20**, 636–642

45. Benton, R. and St Johnston, D. (2003) A conserved oligomerization domain in *Drosophila* Bazooka/PAR-3 is important for apical localization and epithelial polarity. Curr. Biol. **13**, 1330–1334

46. Mizuno, K., Suzuki, A., Hirose, T., Kitamura, K., Kutsuzawa, K., Futaki, M., Amano, Y. and Ohno, S. (2003) Self-association of PAR-3-mediated by the conserved N-terminal domain contributes to the development of epithelial tight junctions. J. Biol. Chem. **278**, 31240–31250

47. Beers, M. and Kemphues, K. (2006) Depletion of the co-chaperone CDC-37 reveals two modes of PAR-6 cortical association in *C. elegans* embryos. Development **133**, 3745–3754

48. Goehring, N.W., Hoege, C., Grill, S.W. and Hyman, A.A. (2011) PAR proteins diffuse freely across the anterior-posterior boundary in polarized *C. elegans* embryos. J. Cell Biol. **193**, 583–594

49. Hao, Y., Boyd, L. and Seydoux, G. (2006) Stabilization of cell polarity by the *C. elegans* RING protein PAR-2. Dev. Cell **10**, 199–208

50. Benton, R. and St Johnston, D. (2003) *Drosophila* PAR-1 and 14-3-3 inhibit Bazooka/PAR-3 to establish complementary cortical domains in polarized cells. Cell **115**, 691–704

51. Hurov, J.B., Watkins, J.L. and Piwnica-Worms, H. (2004) Atypical PKC phosphorylates PAR-1 kinases to regulate localization and activity. Curr. Biol. **14**, 736–741

52. Suzuki, A., Hirata, M., Kamimura, K., Maniwa, R., Yamanaka, T., Mizuno, K., Kishikawa, M., Hirose, H., Amano, Y., Izumi, N. et al. (2004) aPKC acts upstream of PAR-1b in both the establishment and maintenance of mammalian epithelial polarity. Curr. Biol. **14**, 1425–1435

53. Beatty, A., Morton, D. and Kemphues, K. (2010) The *C. elegans* homolog of *Drosophila* lethal giant larvae functions redundantly with PAR-2 to maintain polarity in the early embryo. Development **137**, 3995–4004

54. Hoege, C., Constantinescu, A.T., Schwager, A., Goehring, N.W., Kumar, P. and Hyman, A.A. (2010) LGL can partition the cortex of one-cell *Caenorhabditis elegans* embryos into two domains. Curr. Biol. **20**, 1296–1303

55. Gotta, M., Abraham, M.C. and Ahringer, J. (2001) CDC-42 controls early cell polarity and spindle orientation in *C. elegans*. Curr. Biol. **11**, 482–488

56. Kay, A.J. and Hunter, C.P. (2001) CDC-42 regulates PAR protein localization and function to control cellular and embryonic polarity in *C. elegans*. Curr. Biol. **11**, 474–481

57. Aceto, D., Beers, M. and Kemphues, K.J. (2006) Interaction of PAR-6 with CDC-42 is required for maintenance but not establishment of PAR asymmetry in *C. elegans*. Dev. Biol. **299**, 386–397

58. Hinshaw, J.E. (2000) Dynamin and its role in membrane fission. Annu. Rev. Cell Dev. Biol. **16**, 483–519

59. Nakayama, Y., Shivas, J.M., Poole, D.S., Squirrell, J.M., Kulkoski, J.M., Schleede, J.B. and Skop, A.R. (2009) Dynamin participates in the maintenance of anterior polarity in the *Caenorhabditis elegans* embryo. Dev. Cell **16**, 889–900

60. Schenk, C., Bringmann, H., Hyman, A.A. and Cowan, C.R. (2010) Cortical domain correction repositions the polarity boundary to match the cytokinesis furrow in *C. elegans* embryos. Development **137**, 1743–1753

61. Schubert, C.M., Lin, R., de Vries, C.J., Plasterk, R.H. and Priess, J.R. (2000) MEX-5 and MEX-6 function to establish soma/germline asymmetry in early *C. elegans* embryos. Mol. Cell **5**, 671–682

62. Chase, D., Serafinas, C., Ashcroft, N., Kosinski, M., Longo, D., Ferris, D.K. and Golden, A. (2000) The polo-like kinase PLK-1 is required for nuclear envelope breakdown and the completion of meiosis in *Caenorhabditis elegans*. Genesis **26**, 26–41

63. Nishi, Y., Rogers, E., Robertson, S.M. and Lin, R. (2008) Polo kinases regulate *C. elegans* embryonic polarity via binding to DYRK2-primed MEX-5 and MEX-6. Development **135**, 687–697

64. Budirahardja, Y. and Gonczy, P. (2008) PLK-1 asymmetry contributes to asynchronous cell division of *C. elegans* embryos. Development **135**, 1303–1313

65. Rivers, D.M., Moreno, S., Abraham, M. and Ahringer, J. (2008) PAR proteins direct asymmetry of the cell cycle regulators Polo-like kinase and Cdc25. J. Cell Biol. **180**, 877–885

66. Tabara, H., Hill, R.J., Mello, C.C., Priess, J.R. and Kohara, Y. (1999) pos-1 encodes a cytoplasmic zinc-finger protein essential for germline specification in *C. elegans*. Development **126**, 1–11

67. Reese, K.J., Dunn, M.A., Waddle, J.A. and Seydoux, G. (2000). Asymmetric segregation of PIE-1 in *C. elegans* is mediated by two complementary mechanisms that act through separate PIE-1 protein domains. Mol. Cell **6**, 445–455

68. Tenlen, J.R., Molk, J.N., London, N., Page, B.D. and Priess, J.R. (2008). MEX-5 asymmetry in one-cell *C. elegans* embryos requires PAR-4- and PAR-1-dependent phosphorylation. Development **135**, 3665–3675

69. Daniels, B.R., Perkins, E.M., Dobrowsky, T.M., Sun, S.X. and Wirtz, D. (2009) Asymmetric enrichment of PIE-1 in the *Caenorhabditis elegans* zygote mediated by binary counterdiffusion. J. Cell Biol. **184**, 473–479

70. Daniels, B.R., Dobrowsky, T.M., Perkins, E.M., Sun, S.X. and Wirtz, D. (2010) MEX-5 enrichment in the *C. elegans* early embryo mediated by differential diffusion. Development **137**, 2579–2585

71. Griffin, E.E., Odde, D.J. and Seydoux, G. (2011) Regulation of the MEX-5 gradient by a spatially segregated kinase/phosphatase cycle. Cell **146**, 955–968

72. Batchelder, C., Dunn, M.A., Choy, B., Suh, Y., Cassie, C., Shim, E.Y., Shin, T.H., Mello, C., Seydoux, G. and Blackwell, T.K. (1999) Transcriptional repression by the *Caenorhabditis elegans* germ-line protein PIE-1. Genes Dev. **13**, 202–212

73. Tenenhaus, C., Schubert, C. and Seydoux, G. (1998) Genetic requirements for PIE-1 localization and inhibition of gene expression in the embryonic germ lineage of *Caenorhabditis elegans*. Dev. Biol. **200**, 212–224

74. Budirahardja, Y. and Gonczy, P. (2009) Coupling the cell cycle to development. Development **136**, 2861–2872

75. Noatynska, A., Panbianco, C. and Gotta, M. (2010) SPAT-1/Bora acts with Polo-like kinase 1 to regulate PAR polarity and cell cycle progression. Development **137**, 3315–3325

76. Grill, S.W., Gonczy, P., Stelzer, E.H. and Hyman, A.A. (2001) Polarity controls forces governing asymmetric spindle positioning in the *Caenorhabditis elegans* embryo. Nature **409**, 630–633

77. Morin, X. and Bellaiche, Y. (2011) Mitotic spindle orientation in asymmetric and symmetric cell divisions during animal development. Dev. Cell **21**, 102–119

78. Park, D.H. and Rose, L.S. (2008) Dynamic localization of LIN-5 and GPR-1/2 to cortical force generation domains during spindle positioning. Dev. Biol. **315**, 42–54

79. Labbe, J.C., McCarthy, E.K. and Goldstein, B. (2004) The forces that position a mitotic spindle asymmetrically are tethered until after the time of spindle assembly. J. Cell Biol. **167**, 245–256

80. Panbianco, C., Weinkove, D., Zanin, E., Jones, D., Divecha, N., Gotta, M. and Ahringer, J. (2008) A casein kinase 1 and PAR proteins regulate asymmetry of a PIP$_2$ synthesis enzyme for asymmetric spindle positioning. Dev. Cell **15**, 198–208

81. Galli, M., Munoz, J., Portegijs, V., Boxem, M., Grill, S.W., Heck, A.J. and van den Heuvel, S. (2011) aPKC phosphorylates NuMA-related LIN-5 to position the mitotic spindle during asymmetric division. Nat. Cell Biol. **13**, 1132–1138

82. Schneider, S.Q. and Bowerman, B. (2003) Cell polarity and the cytoskeleton in the *Caenorhabditis elegans* zygote. Annu. Rev. Genet. **37**, 221–249

© The Authors Journal compilation © 2012 Biochemical Society
Essays Biochem. (2012) **53**, 15–27: doi: 10.1042/BSE0530015

2

Phosphoinositide lipids and cell polarity: linking the plasma membrane to the cytocortex

Michael P. Krahn[*][†] and Andreas Wodarz[*][1]

Stem Cell Biology, Department of Anatomy and Cell Biology, Georg-August-University Göttingen, Justus-von-Liebig-Weg 11, 37077 Göttingen, Germany, and †Institute for Molecular and Cellular Anatomy, University of Regensburg, Universitätsstr. 31, 93053 Regensburg, Germany

Abstract

Many cell types in animals and plants are polarized, which means that the cell is subdivided into functionally and structurally distinct compartments. Epithelial cells, for example, possess an apical side facing a lumen or the outside environment and a basolateral side facing adjacent epithelial cells and the basement membrane. Neurons possess distinct axonal and dendritic compartments with specific functions in sending and receiving signals. Migrating cells form a leading edge that actively engages in pathfinding and cell-substrate attachment, and a trailing edge where such attachments are abandoned. In all of these cases, both the plasma membrane and the cytocortex directly underneath the plasma membrane show differences in their molecular composition and structural organization. In this chapter we will focus on a specific type of membrane lipids, the phosphoinositides, because in polarized cells they show a polarized distribution

[1]*To whom correspondence should be addressed (email awodarz@gwdg.de).*

in the plasma membrane. They furthermore influence the molecular organization of the cytocortex by recruiting specific protein binding partners which are involved in the regulation of the cytoskeleton and in signal transduction cascades that control polarity, growth and cell migration.

Introduction

The functional compartmentalization of a polarized cell can be nicely illustrated in the case of a typical epithelial cell, for instance a cell of the small intestine (Figure 1). The major function of this cell type is the uptake of nutrients from the food that passes through the lumen of the gut. The apical plasma membrane of the gut epithelial cell is in direct contact with the food in the gut lumen and possesses numerous transporters and ion channels for glucose, amino acids, lipids and other important substances that have to be extracted from the food. To facilitate the uptake of substances from the food, the apical surface of the gut epithelial

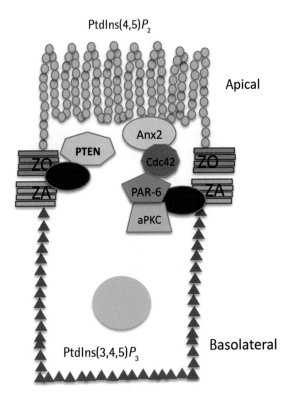

Figure 1. Polarized localization of PtdIns(4,5)P_2 and PtdIns(3,4,5)P_3 in mammalian epithelial cells
PtdIns(4,5)P_2 (circles) is enriched in the apical plasma membrane domain, whereas PtdIns(3,4,5)P_3 (triangles) is confined to the basolateral plasma membrane. PAR-3 is localized to the junctional region, where it interacts with the other components of the PAR complex and with PTEN. Annexin 2 (Anx2) binds directly to PtdIns(4,5)P_2 in the apical plasma membrane.

cells is enormously enlarged by the formation of microvilli, finger-like protrusions of the plasma membrane that are formed by a specialized arrangement of actin filaments directly underneath the membrane in the apical cytocortex. On the other hand, the basolateral plasma membrane of the gut epithelial cells is engaged in the formation of various types of intercellular junctions (Figure 1). The most apical of these junctions is the tight junction, also called ZO (zonula occludens), which forms a diffusion barrier between the apical and the basolateral plasma membrane domains and seals the intercellular space to prevent leakage of small molecules and water between the epithelial cells. Basally to the tight junction the ZA (zonula adherens) is formed, an adhesion belt composed of cadherins and catenins, which is closely linked to the cortical actin cytoskeleton. From this example it is obvious that the protein composition of the plasma membrane differs between the apical and the basolateral plasma membrane domain, and that the different composition of the membrane is reflected in a different organization of the cytocortex. In the following paragraphs we will discuss how the polarized localization of phosphoinositide membrane lipids links the polarity of the plasma membrane to the organization of the cytocortex.

Phosphoinositides as components of biological membranes

The core of the plasma membrane is formed by a bilayer of phospholipids. One of the major classes of phospholipids in biological membranes are glycerophospholipids, consisting of a glycerol moiety esterified with two fatty acid chains that protrude into the centre of the lipid bilayer and a polar head group that faces the cytosol or the extracellular space and is linked to the glycerol moiety via a phosphate group.

The polar head group of a class of glycerophospholipids, called phosphoinositides, is the cyclic alcohol inositol that can be phosphorylated at the hydroxy groups 3, 4 and 5 in seven possible combinations (Figure 2). Phosphoinositides are exclusively localized on the cytosolic face of biological membranes and show a strong specificity with respect to their distribution in different membrane compartments. PtdIns$3P$ is enriched in endosomal membranes, whereas PtdIns$4P$ is enriched in membranes of the Golgi apparatus and in the plasma membrane. In this chapter, however, we will focus on PtdIns(4,5)P_2 and PtdIns(3,4,5)P_3, two phosphoinositides that are commonly present in the cytosolic face of the plasma membrane and are important regulators of cell polarity. PtdIns(4,5)P_2 was first identified as a substrate for PLC (phospholipase C). Upon stimulation of many GPCRs (G-protein-coupled receptors), activated PLC selectively binds to PtdIns(4,5)P_2 and cleaves it into DAG (diacylglycerol) and Ins(1,4,5)P_3 [1–3], which both serve as second messengers for various intracellular signalling cascades.

By the action of a number of specific kinases and phosphatases, phosphoinositides are dynamically modified or converted into other phosphoinositides by phosphorylation and dephosphorylation reactions. PtdIns(4,5)P_2

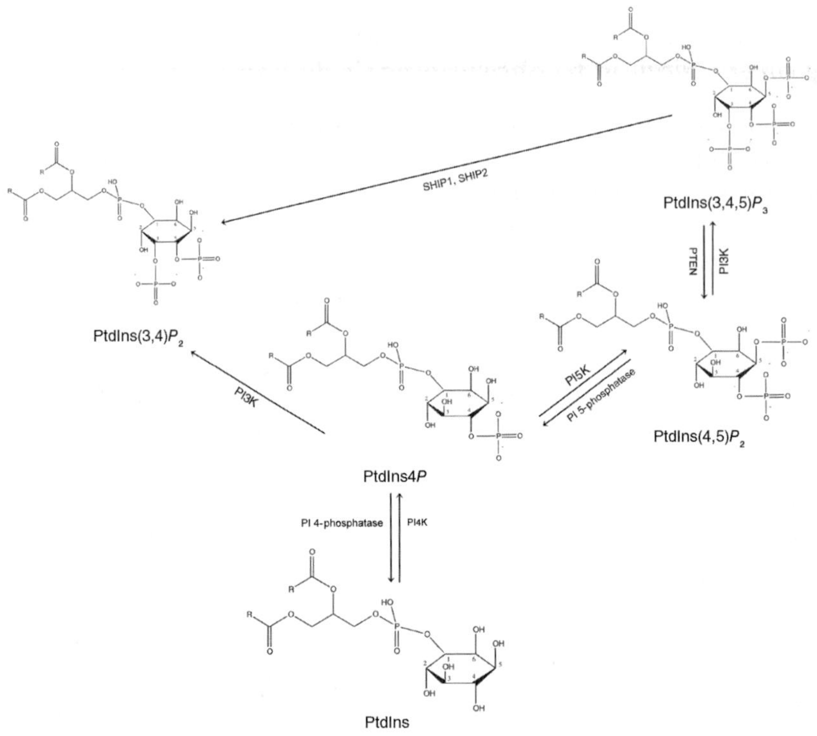

Figure 2. Phosphoinositides implicated in the control of cell polarity
The structure of the phosphoinositides discussed in the present chapter. The names of the enzymes that convert one phosphoinositide into another one are given next to the arrows. R, fatty acid esterified with the glycerol backbone of the phosphoinositides. SHIP, SH2 (Src homology 2)-domain-containing inositol phosphatase.

is synthesized from PtdIns in two steps. First the PI4K (phosphoinositide 4-kinase) converts PtdIns into PtdIns4P. Subsequently, the plasma-membrane-associated PI5K (phosphoinositide 5-kinase) phosphorylates the hydroxy group at position 5 of the inositol ring to produce PtdIns(4,5)P_2 [4]. Only a small fraction of PtdIns(4,5)P_2 gets phosphorylated by class I PI3Ks (phosphoinositide 3-kinases) to produce PtdIns(3,4,5)P_3 [5]. This catalytic step is highly regulated and is triggered by activation of class I PI3Ks via the stimulation of a number of cell-surface receptors, including growth factor receptors, e.g. by insulin, growth hormone, nerve growth factor and epidermal growth factor [6]. Class I PI3Ks are antagonized by the PTEN (phosphatase and tensin homologue) phosphatase, which removes the phosphate from position 3 of the inositol ring [7]. Although several phosphoinositides are substrates for class I PI3Ks and PTEN, the phosphorylation of PtdIns(4,5)P_2 at position 3 by PI3K to generate PtdIns(3,4,5)P_3 and the corresponding dephosphorylation of PtdIns(3,4,5)P_3 by PTEN to generate PtdIns(4,5)P_2 are the most relevant modifications of phosphoinositides in the context of this chapter.

Recruitment of cytosolic proteins to biological membranes by direct binding to phosphoinositide head groups

Owing to their localization in the cytosolic leaflet of biological membranes and because their production and turnover can be spatially and temporally regulated, phosphoinositides are ideally suited to recruit cytosolic proteins to specific membrane compartments. This is important for the activation of many enzymes, including kinases and phosphatases, and for the proper assembly of the cytoskeleton in the cytocortex. The interaction of cytosolic proteins with phosphoinositides is mediated by selective lipid-binding domains that are able to discriminate between the different phosphoinositides. Well-known examples for such domains are the PH (pleckstrin homology), PX (phagocyte oxidase homology) and FYVE domains (see Table 1). A direct interaction of either

Table 1. Proteins and identified protein domains which directly bind to lipids within biological membranes

Protein name	Lipid-binding domain	Specificity	Function
Pleckstrin	PH	PtdIns$(4,5)P_2$	Activation of platelets
Phosphoinositide PLC (δ, β, γ, ε, ζ, η)	PH	PtdIns$(4,5)P_2$	Generation of second messengers [Ins$(1,4,5)P_3$ and DAG] by cleavage of PtdIns$(4,5)P_2$ upon activation
Akt (PKB)	PH	PtdIns$(3,4)P_2$ and PtdIns$(3,4,5)P_3$	Activator of various signalling pathways
PDK1	PH	PtdIns$(3,4)P_2$ and PtdIns$(3,4,5)P_3$	Activation of several kinases
p47^{phox}	PX	PtdIns3P	Activation of phagocyte oxidase
PKC	C1	DAG	Activator of various signalling pathways
PKC	C2	Acidic phospholipids	Activator of various signalling pathways
Phospholipase A$_2$, phospholipase δ1	C2 (+Ca^{2+})	Acidic phospholipids	Cleavage of phospholipids
Endosomal proteins [e.g. Vps27p (vacuolar protein sorting 27p), EEA1 (early endosome antigen 1)]	FYVE (+Zn^{2+})	PtdIns3P	Endosomal localization of proteins
Epsin	ENTH (epsin N-terminal homology)	PtdIns$(4,5)P_2$	Enodcytic clathrin adaptors

one of these complex folded domains or of only a stretch of positively charged (basic) amino acids within a cytosolic protein with phosphoinositides has been described for a large number of proteins. In a proteomic approach, Catimel et al. [8] pulled down 388 proteins from mammalian cell extracts with PtdIns(3,5)P_2- and PtdIns(4,5)P_2-coated beads [8]. Even in the absence of a defined phospho-inositide-binding domain or a contiguous stretch of basic amino acids, some proteins are capable of directly binding to phosphoinositides in the plasma membrane. Several basic amino acids which might be scattered over a longer distance within the linear protein sequence are sufficient for binding to PtdIns(4,5)P_2 and PtdIns(3,4,5)P_3 [9]. By three-dimensional protein folding, these residues come together to form a positively charged pocket for the acidic head groups of the phosphoinositides.

Proteins mediating downstream effects of phosphoinositides

Local accumulation of PtdIns(4,5)P_2 and PtdIns(3,4,5)P_3 in specific regions of the plasma membrane results in the recruitment of certain proteins containing the corresponding lipid-binding domains. For one of these proteins, PDK1 (phosphoinositide-dependent kinase 1), a function as a master activator of various intracellular signal transduction pathways has been demonstrated [10]. PDK1 is a constitutively active kinase that directly binds to PtdIns(3,4,5)P_3 and PtdIns(3,4)P_2 via its PH domain. Among the phosphorylation targets of PDK1 are classical, as well as atypical, PKC (protein kinase C; aPKC is atypical PKC) isoforms [11,12] and the kinase Akt [also known as PKB (protein kinase B)] [10]. Like PDK1, Akt contains a PH domain specific for PtdIns(3,4,5)P_3 and PtdIns(3,4)P_2 [13,14] which is responsible for targeting Akt to the plasma membrane in the vicinity of its activating kinase PDK1. In addition, PtdIns(3,4,5)P_3 induces a conformational change in Akt that allows its phosphorylation by PDK1 [15]. Thus the activation of Akt by PDK1 is regulated at the level of substrate recruitment to the plasma membrane and PtdIns(3,4,5)P_3-dependent changes in substrate conformation rather than by activation of the upstream kinase PDK1 [16].

Activated Akt dissociates from the plasma membrane and phosphorylates numerous targets in the cytosol and in the nucleus, among them key regulators of pivotal cellular processes such as apoptosis/survival, cell-cycle control, glucose metabolism, cell migration and cell proliferation [17]. Thus overabundance of PtdIns(3,4,5)P_3 in the plasma membrane, caused either by hyperactivation of the PI3K pathway or by loss-of-function of PTEN, is a frequent cause of cancer and Type II diabetes mediated by Akt signalling.

Phosphoinositides control the polarity of migrating cells

The polarized distribution of PtdIns(4,5)P_2 and PtdIns(3,4,5)P_3 is an ancient evolutionarily conserved mechanism to control cell polarity and cytoskeleton rearrangements in many migratory cell types. Migrating cells of the slime mould *Dictyostelium discoideum* accumulate active PI3K at the plasma membrane of the leading edge facing a chemoattractant, whereas PTEN localizes at the side and the rear of the cell [18,19]. It has been proposed that this complementary localization of PI3K and PTEN, which causes a corresponding polarity in the localization of PtdIns(4,5)P_2 and PtdIns(3,4,5)P_3 in the plasma membrane, serves to translate the very small differences in the extracellular concentration of the chemoattractant into a steeper intracellular gradient of binding sites for regulators of the cortical actin cytoskeleton [20]. Indeed, gain- and loss-of-function of both PI3K and PTEN disrupt polarity and cytoskeleton rearrangements in migrating *Dictyostelium*.

Essentially the same mechanism appears to operate in human white blood cells, called neutrophils, during migration. PtdIns(3,4,5)P_3 is enriched at the leading edge, whereas PtdIns(4,5)P_2 is excluded from the leading edge. Furthermore, pseudopod formation, which is crucial for directed movement, depends on PtdIns(3,4,5)P_3 accumulation at the leading edge [21,22]. Notably, enrichment of PtdIns(3,4,5)P_3 results in a positive-feedback loop leading to increased local accumulation of PtdIns(3,4,5)P_3, which depends on PI3K and Rho GTPases.

In 1998 Tamura et al. [23] reported that, in mouse fibroblasts, loss of PTEN results in increased cell motility, whereas overexpression of PTEN inhibits cell motility. This was confirmed by Liliental et al. [24] who showed that the activity of Rac1 and Cdc42 (cell division cycle 42) was increased upon loss of PTEN, and that expression of dominant-negative versions of these small GTPases abolished the PTEN loss-of-function phenotype [24]. Together, these data clearly indicate that the polarized distribution of PtdIns(4,5)P_2 and PtdIns(3,4,5)P_3 in migrating cells leads to local differences in the organization of the actin cytoskeleton which are essential for protrusion formation and directional cell movement.

Phosphoinositides control the polarity of non-migratory cells

PtdIns(3,4,5)P_3 has also been implicated in the polarization of hippocampal neurons. One of the earliest markers of the single neurite that is going to become the axon is the accumulation of PI3K and Akt, which directly binds to PtdIns(3,4,5)P_3. Overexpression of PTEN or inhibition of PI3K abolishes polarization of hippocampal neurons, pointing to an essential function of PtdIns(3,4,5)P_3 in determining the axon [25].

In a three-dimensional cyst model of polarizing mammalian epithelial cells, PtdIns(4,5)P_2 is enriched at the apical plasma membrane, whereas PtdIns(3,4,5)P_3 is confined to the basolateral membrane [26]. PTEN localizes to the apical plasma membrane and functions to segregate PtdIns(4,5)P_2 from PtdIns(3,4,5)P_3. This polarized distribution of phosphoinositides apparently functions as a polarity cue, because PtdIns(4,5)P_2 ectopically delivered to the basolateral membrane recruits the apical determinant annexin 2, which in turn leads to mislocalization of Cdc42 to the lateral plasma membrane. Cdc42 in turn is a central regulator of actin polymerization that controls the dynamic rearrangements of the cytoskeleton in polarized cells. Since loss of Cdc42 function results in impaired cyst formation, taken together these findings indicate that the apical recruitment of the annexin 2–Cdc42 complex by PtdIns(4,5)P_2 is crucial for cyst formation. Consistent with this model, depletion of PTEN results in the unpolarized distribution of PtdIns(4,5)P_2, PtdIns(3,4,5)P_3 and annexin 2, which prevents proper lumen formation [26].

The reverse approach pursued by Gassama-Diagne et al. [27] underlines the importance of the differential localization of phosphatidylinositol phosphates for the determination of the apical versus the basolateral plasma membrane domains [27]. The authors produced ectopic patches of basolateral plasma membrane by introduction of PtdIns(3,4,5)P_3 into the apical plasma membrane. These patches formed protrusions that contained membrane proteins normally only present in the basolateral membrane and excluded apical proteins. Inhibition of PI3K by a specific inhibitor decreased the size of the lateral plasma membrane and overall cell height. Blocking endocytosis by expression of a dominant-negative dynamin abolished the formation of basolateral protrusions in the apical membrane domain, indicating that PtdIns(3,4,5)P_3 present in the apical plasma membrane is capable of redirecting endocytosed vesicles containing basolateral membrane proteins to ectopic sites. Taken together, these data convincingly show that the ectopic insertion of PtdIns(3,4,5)P_3 into the apical plasma membrane confers basolateral properties on this patch of membrane.

An important question in this context is how plasma membrane polarity, cytoskeleton organization and endocytic trafficking are connected to each other. There is now increasing evidence that this link may be provided by the small Rho GTPases Cdc42 and Rac. Cdc42 and Rac were shown to associate with and activate PI3K [28–30]. Vice versa, PtdIns(3,4,5)P_3 directly activates two GEFs (guanine-nucleotide-exchange factors), which promote Rac activity [31,32]. Furthermore, the activity of one of these GEFs is inhibited by PtdIns(4,5)P_2 [32]. Thus recruitment and activation of Rac by PtdIns(3,4,5)P_3 directly and via Rac-specific GEFs appears to provide an efficient mechanism to locally modulate the actin cytoskeleton in migrating cells and epithelial cells. The situation is not as clear for Cdc42, since it can be recruited by both PtdIns(4,5)P_2 and PtdIns(3,4,5)P_3 [26,27]. Thus the existence of additional regulatory mechanisms has been postulated that either influence Cdc42 activity or function downstream of Cdc42 in the control of cell polarity [33].

Interactions between phosphoinositides and PAR (PARtitioning defective) proteins

One important link between Cdc42 and the regulation of cell polarity is provided by the PAR-3–PAR-6–aPKC complex. This protein complex, named the

PAR complex below, is a key regulator of cell polarity in many different cell types throughout the animal kingdom [34,35]. Cdc42 binds directly to PAR-6, a core component of the PAR complex [36–38]. The biochemical interaction between Cdc42 and the PAR complex is essential for Rac activation downstream of Cdc42, leading to rearrangements of the cytoskeleton followed by neurite growth and axon specification [39]. In mammalian cultured neurons, localization of PAR-3 at the tip of the axon depends on PtdIns(3,4,5)P_3 and PI3K [25]. Overexpression of PAR-3 or PAR-6 resulted in impaired axon determination, leaving cells with two or more axon-like neurites. In *Caenorhabditis elegans*, the localization of the PAR complex is dependent on Cdc42 activity, either due to the direct interaction of Cdc42 with PAR-6 or indirectly via the impact of Cdc42 on the cytoskeleton [40,41]. Thus the PtdIns(3,4,5)P_3–Cdc42 connection appears to be an ancient mechanism to restrict the localization and/or the activity of the PAR complex.

Recent work has revealed a direct interaction between one of the PAR proteins, PAR-3, called Baz (Bazooka) in the fruit fly, and phosphoinositides. We have shown that Baz directly binds to PtdIns(4,5)P_2 and PtdIns(3,4,5)P_3 via a stretch of basic amino acid residues at its C-terminal region [42] and this finding was confirmed for mammalian PAR-3 [43]. For many proteins containing polybasic lipid-binding domains similar to the one in Baz it was shown that the depletion of only PtdIns(4,5)P_2 or PtdIns(3,4,5)P_3 does not affect their cortical localization [9]. Only if both phosphoinositides are depleted do these proteins accumulate in the cytoplasm. The promiscuity in phosphoinositide binding allows recruitment of Baz to the cortex, even in unpolarized cells, prior to the formation of cell–cell junctions and the establishment of cell polarity. This is consistent with Baz being one of the earliest regulators of cell polarity, which is required for triggering the segregation of PtdIns(4,5)P_2 and PtdIns(3,4,5)P_3 into different plasma membrane domains upon full polarization of the cell.

How could Baz/PAR-3 promote the segregation of PtdIns(4,5)P_2 and PtdIns(3,4,5)P_3 in the plasma membrane upon cell polarization? We have previously demonstrated that Baz directly binds to PTEN and recruits it to the apical junctional region in epithelial cells [44]. In *Drosophila* photoreceptor cells, Baz-dependent targeting of PTEN to the ZA is crucial for PtdIns(3,4,5)P_3 accumulation in a specialized apical domain of the plasma membrane [45]. In the polarizing ectodermal epithelium of *Drosophila* embryos, loss of Baz function abolishes the proper junctional localization of the synaptotagmin-like protein Bitesize, which directly binds to PtdIns(4,5)P_2 [46]. The interaction of PAR-3 with PTEN has been confirmed in mammalian MDCK (Madin–Darby canine kidney) cells and was shown to be essential for proper establishment of polarity [47,48]. Together with the finding that depletion of PTEN abolishes polarization of three-dimensional cysts of MDCK cells [26], recruitment of PTEN by Baz/PAR-3 can now be considered an essential functional step in plasma membrane polarization.

Manipulation of phosphoinositide signalling by bacterial pathogens

A fascinating twist to the function of phosphoinositides in cell polarity is their manipulation by bacterial pathogens in order to facilitate the entry of bacteria into the cell. *Salmonella* expresses a PtdIns 4-phosphatase that hydrolyses PtdIns(4,5)P_2 to PtdIns5P. Loss of PtdIns(4,5)P_2 from the apical plasma membrane leads to rearrangement of the cytoskeleton and the loss of the tight junctions [49]. This breakdown of epithelial integrity allows the bacterium to overwhelm the epithelial barrier. Another bacterium, *Pseudomonas aeruginosa*, penetrates epithelial cells more efficiently through the basolateral plasma membrane than through the apical membrane domain. However, attachment of the pathogen to the apical plasma membrane induces focal accumulation of PI3K and PtdIns(3,4,5)P_3, as well as re-localization of basolateral markers, facilitating infection of the cell by *P. aeruginosa* [50,51].

Conclusion

Phosphoinositides are membrane lipids that are unique with respect to their compartmentalized localization in the cell. In the context of cell polarity, PtdIns(4,5)P_2 and PtdIns(3,4,5)P_3 show a mutually exclusive localization in the plasma membrane and recruit specific binding partners to the cortex that control the organization of the cytoskeleton and various intracellular signalling pathways. On the other hand, polarity regulators, including the PAR complex, contribute to the polarized localization of phosphoinositides in the plasma membrane by localized recruitment of the lipid phosphatase PTEN. Together, phosphoinositides, PAR proteins and regulators of the cytoskeleton, in particular the small GTPases Rac and Cdc42, form a complex network of interactions that controls the polarized phenotype of many different cell types.

Summary

- *Phosphoinositides are always localized on the cytosolic face of biological membranes.*
- *Different phosphoinositides are enriched in specific subcellular membrane compartments.*
- *Phosphoinositides recruit cortical proteins via specific phosphoinositide-binding domains.*
- *PtdIns(4,5)P_2 and PtdIns(3,4,5)P_3 show a polarized and mutually exclusive localization in the plasma membrane of migratory cells, epithelia and other polarized cell types.*
- *PtdIns(4,5)P_2 and PtdIns(3,4,5)P_3 are functionally linked to proteins of the PAR complex and to the small GTPases Rac and Cdc42.*

- *Some bacterial pathogens manipulate the phosphoinositide composition of the plasma membrane to gain entry into the cell.*

The work of the authors is supported by the Forschungsförderprogramm of the University Medicine Göttingen (to M.P.K.) and by the Deutsche Forschungsgemeinschaft [grant numbers KR 390/1-1 (to M.P.K.), and grant numbers SFB 523, SFB 590, SPP 1109, SPP 1111, FOR 942, FOR 1756, DFG Research Center Molecular Physiology of the Brain) (to A.W.)].

References

1. Berridge, M.J. and Irvine, R.F. (1984) Inositol trisphosphate, a novel second messenger in cellular signal transduction. Nature **312**, 315–321
2. Kirk, C.J., Bone, E.A., Palmer, S. and Michell, R.H. (1984) The role of phosphatidylinositol 4,5 bisphosphate breakdown in cell-surface receptor activation. J. Recept. Res. **4**, 489–504
3. Smrcka, A.V., Hepler, J.R., Brown, K.O. and Sternweis, P.C. (1991) Regulation of polyphosphoinositide-specific phospholipase C activity by purified Gq. Science **251**, 804–807
4. Mao, Y.S. and Yin, H.L. (2007) Regulation of the actin cytoskeleton by phosphatidylinositol 4-phosphate 5 kinases. Pflügers Arch. **455**, 5–18
5. Auger, K.R., Serunian, L.A., Soltoff, S.P., Libby, P. and Cantley, L.C. (1989) PDGF-dependent tyrosine phosphorylation stimulates production of novel polyphosphoinositides in intact cells. Cell **57**, 167–175
6. Cantley, L.C. (2002) The phosphoinositide 3-kinase pathway. Science **296**, 1655–1657
7. Downes, C.P., Bennett, D., McConnachie, G., Leslie, N.R., Pass, I., MacPhee, C., Patel, L. and Gray, A. (2001) Antagonism of PI 3-kinase-dependent signalling pathways by the tumour suppressor protein, PTEN. Biochem. Soc. Trans. **29**, 846–851
8. Catimel, B., Schieber, C., Condron, M., Patsiouras, H., Connolly, L., Catimel, J., Nice, E.C., Burgess, A.W. and Holmes, A.B. (2008) The PI(3,5)P2 and PI(4,5)P2 interactomes. J. Proteome Res. **7**, 5295–5313
9. Heo, W.D., Inoue, T., Park, W.S., Kim, M.L., Park, B.O., Wandless, T.J. and Meyer, T. (2006) PI(3,4,5)P3 and PI(4,5)P2 lipids target proteins with polybasic clusters to the plasma membrane. Science **314**, 1458–1461
10. Alessi, D.R., James, S.R., Downes, C.P., Holmes, A.B., Gaffney, P.R., Reese, C.B. and Cohen, P. (1997) Characterization of a 3-phosphoinositide-dependent protein kinase which phosphorylates and activates protein kinase Bα. Curr. Biol. **7**, 261–269
11. Le Good, J.A., Ziegler, W.H., Parekh, D.B., Alessi, D.R., Cohen, P. and Parker, P.J. (1998) Protein kinase C isotypes controlled by phosphoinositide 3-kinase through the protein kinase PDK1. Science **281**, 2042–2045
12. Nakanishi, H., Brewer, K.A. and Exton, J.H. (1993) Activation of the zeta isozyme of protein kinase C by phosphatidylinositol 3,4,5-trisphosphate. J. Biol. Chem. **268**, 13–16
13. James, S.R., Downes, C.P., Gigg, R., Grove, S.J., Holmes, A.B. and Alessi, D.R. (1996) Specific binding of the Akt-1 protein kinase to phosphatidylinositol 3,4,5-trisphosphate without subsequent activation. Biochem. J. **315**, 709–713
14. Franke, T.F., Kaplan, D.R., Cantley, L.C. and Toker, A. (1997) Direct regulation of the Akt proto-oncogene product by phosphatidylinositol-3,4-bisphosphate. Science **275**, 665–668
15. Stokoe, D., Stephens, L.R., Copeland, T., Gaffney, P.R., Reese, C.B., Painter, G.F., Holmes, A.B., McCormick, F. and Hawkins, P.T. (1997) Dual role of phosphatidylinositol-3,4,5-trisphosphate in the activation of protein kinase B. Science **277**, 567–570

16. Mora, A., Komander, D., van Aalten, D.M. and Alessi, D.R. (2004) PDK1, the master regulator of AGC kinase signal transduction. Semin. Cell Dev. Biol. **15**, 161–170

17. Woodgett, J.R. (2005) Recent advances in the protein kinase B signaling pathway. Curr. Opin. Cell Biol. **17**, 150–157

18. Funamoto, S., Meili, R., Lee, S., Parry, L. and Firtel, R.A. (2002) Spatial and temporal regulation of 3-phosphoinositides by PI 3-kinase and PTEN mediates chemotaxis. Cell **109**, 611–623

19. Iijima, M. and Devreotes, P. (2002) Tumor suppressor PTEN mediates sensing of chemoattractant gradients. Cell **109**, 599–610

20. Charest, P.G. and Firtel, R.A. (2006) Feedback signaling controls leading-edge formation during chemotaxis. Curr. Opin. Genet. Dev. **16**, 339–347

21. Wang, F., Herzmark, P., Weiner, O.D., Srinivasan, S., Servant, G. and Bourne, H.R. (2002) Lipid products of PI(3)Ks maintain persistent cell polarity and directed motility in neutrophils. Nat. Cell Biol. **4**, 513–518

22. Weiner, O.D., Neilsen, P.O., Prestwich, G.D., Kirschner, M.W., Cantley, L.C. and Bourne, H.R. (2002) A PtdInsP(3)- and Rho GTPase-mediated positive feedback loop regulates neutrophil polarity. Nat. Cell Biol. **4**, 509–513

23. Tamura, M., Gu, J., Matsumoto, K., Aota, S., Parsons, R. and Yamada, K.M. (1998) Inhibition of cell migration, spreading, and focal adhesions by tumor suppressor PTEN. Science **280**, 1614–1617

24. Liliental, J., Moon, S.Y., Lesche, R., Mamillapalli, R., Li, D., Zheng, Y., Sun, H. and Wu, H. (2000) Genetic deletion of the Pten tumor suppressor gene promotes cell motility by activation of Rac1 and Cdc42 GTPases. Curr. Biol. **10**, 401–404

25. Shi, S.H., Jan, L.Y. and Jan, Y.N. (2003) Hippocampal neuronal polarity specified by spatially localized mPar3/mPar6 and PI 3-kinase activity. Cell **112**, 63–75

26. Martin-Belmonte, F., Gassama, A., Datta, A., Yu, W., Rescher, U., Gerke, V. and Mostov, K. (2007) PTEN-mediated apical segregation of phosphoinositides controls epithelial morphogenesis through Cdc42. Cell **128**, 383–397

27. Gassama-Diagne, A., Yu, W., ter Beest, M., Martin-Belmonte, F., Kierbel, A., Engel, J. and Mostov, K. (2006) Phosphatidylinositol-3,4,5-trisphosphate regulates the formation of the basolateral plasma membrane in epithelial cells. Nat. Cell Biol. **8**, 963–970

28. Tolias, K.F., Cantley, L.C. and Carpenter, C.L. (1995) Rho family GTPases bind to phosphoinositide kinases. J. Biol. Chem. **270**, 17656–17659

29. Keely, P.J., Westwick, J.K., Whitehead, I.P., Der, C.J. and Parise, L.V. (1997) Cdc42 and Rac1 induce integrin-mediated cell motility and invasiveness through PI(3)K. Nature **390**, 632–636

30. Chan, T.O., Rodeck, U., Chan, A.M., Kimmelman, A.C., Rittenhouse, S.E., Panayotou, G. and Tsichlis, P.N. (2002) Small GTPases and tyrosine kinases coregulate a molecular switch in the phosphoinositide 3-kinase regulatory subunit. Cancer Cell **1**, 181–191

31. Welch, H.C., Coadwell, W.J., Ellson, C.D., Ferguson, G.J., Andrews, S.R., Erdjument-Bromage, H., Tempst, P., Hawkins, P.T. and Stephens, L.R. (2002) P-Rex1, a PtdIns(3,4,5)P3- and Gβγ-regulated guanine-nucleotide exchange factor for Rac. Cell **108**, 809–821

32. Han, J., Luby-Phelps, K., Das, B., Shu, X., Xia, Y., Mosteller, R.D., Krishna, U.M., Falck, J.R., White, M.A. and Broek, D. (1998) Role of substrates and products of PI 3-kinase in regulating activation of Rac-related guanosine triphosphatases by Vav. Science **279**, 558–560

33. Gassama-Diagne, A. and Payrastre, B. (2009) Phosphoinositide signaling pathways: promising role as builders of epithelial cell polarity. Int. Rev. Cell Mol. Biol. **273**, 313–343

34. Suzuki, A. and Ohno, S. (2006) The PAR-aPKC system: lessons in polarity. J. Cell Sci. **119**, 979–987

35. Goldstein, B. and Macara, I.G. (2007) The PAR proteins: fundamental players in animal cell polarization. Dev. Cell **13**, 609–622

36. Joberty, G., Petersen, C., Gao, L. and Macara, I.G. (2000) The cell-polarity protein Par6 links Par3 and atypical protein kinase C to Cdc42. Nat. Cell Biol. **2**, 531–539

37. Johansson, A., Driessens, M. and Aspenstrom, P. (2000) The mammalian homologue of the *Caenorhabditis elegans* polarity protein PAR-6 is a binding partner for the Rho GTPases cdc42 and racl. J. Cell Sci. **113**, 3267–3275

38. Lin, D., Edwards, A.S., Fawcett, J.P., Mbamalu, G., Scott, J.D. and Pawson, T. (2000) A mammalian Par-3-Par-6 complex implicated in CdC42/Racl and aPKC signalling and cell polarity. Nat. Cell Biol. **2**, 540–547

39. Nishimura, T., Yamaguchi, T., Kato, K., Yoshizawa, M., Nabeshima, Y., Ohno, S., Hoshino, M. and Kaibuchi, K. (2005) PAR-6-PAR-3 mediates Cdc42-induced Rac activation through the Rac GEFs STEF/Tiaml. Nat. Cell Biol. **7**, 270–277

40. Gotta, M., Abraham, M.C. and Ahringer, J. (2001) CDC-42 controls early cell polarity and spindle orientation in *C. elegans*. Curr. Biol. **11**, 482–488

41. Kay, A.J. and Hunter, C.P. (2001) CDC-42 regulates PAR protein localization and function to control cellular and embryonic polarity in *C. elegans*. Curr. Biol. **11**, 474–481

42. Krahn, M.P., Klopfenstein, D.R., Fischer, N. and Wodarz, A. (2010) Membrane targeting of Bazooka/PAR-3 is mediated by direct binding to phosphoinositide lipids. Curr. Biol. **20**, 636–642

43. Horikoshi, Y., Hamada, S., Ohno, S. and Suetsugu, S. (2011) Phosphoinositide binding by par-3 involved in par-3 localization. Cell Struct. Funct. **36**, 97–102

44. von Stein, W., Ramrath, A., Grimm, A., Muller-Borg, M. and Wodarz, A. (2005) Direct association of Bazooka/PAR-3 with the lipid phosphatase PTEN reveals a link between the PAR/aPKC complex and phosphoinositide signaling. Development **132**, 1675–1686

45. Pinal, N., Goberdhan, D.C., Collinson, L., Fujita, Y., Cox, I.M., Wilson, C. and Pichaud, F. (2006) Regulated and polarized PtdIns(3,4,5)P3 accumulation is essential for apical membrane morphogenesis in photoreceptor epithelial cells. Curr. Biol. **16**, 140–149

46. Pilot, F., Philippe, J.M., Lemmers, C. and Lecuit, T. (2006) Spatial control of actin organization at adherens junctions by a synaptotagmin-like protein Btsz. Nature **442**, 580–584

47. Feng, W., Wu, H., Chan, L.N. and Zhang, M. (2008) Par-3-mediated junctional localization of the lipid phosphatase PTEN is required for cell polarity establishment. J. Biol. Chem. **283**, 23440–23449

48. Wu, H., Feng, W., Chen, J., Chan, L.N., Huang, S. and Zhang, M. (2007) PDZ domains of Par-3 as potential phosphoinositide signaling integrators. Mol. Cell **28**, 886–898

49. Mason, D., Mallo, G.V., Terebiznik, M.R., Payrastre, B., Finlay, B.B., Brumell, J.H., Rameh, L. and Grinstein, S. (2007) Alteration of epithelial structure and function associated with PtdIns(4,5)P2 degradation by a bacterial phosphatase. J. Gen. Physiol. **129**, 267–283

50. Kierbel, A., Gassama-Diagne, A., Rocha, C., Radoshevich, L., Olson, J., Mostov, K. and Engel, J. (2007) *Pseudomonas aeruginosa* exploits a PIP3-dependent pathway to transform apical into basolateral membrane. J. Cell Biol. **177**, 21–27

51. Kierbel, A., Gassama-Diagne, A., Mostov, K. and Engel, J.N. (2005) The phosphoinositol-3-kinase-protein kinase B/Akt pathway is critical for *Pseudomonas aeruginosa* strain PAK internalization. Mol. Biol. Cell **16**, 2577–2585

© The Authors Journal compilation © 2012 Biochemical Society
Essays Biochem. (2012) **53**, 29–39 doi: 10.1042/BSE0530029

3

The role of secretory and endocytic pathways in the maintenance of cell polarity

Su Fen Ang and Heike Fölsch[1]

Department of Cell and Molecular Biology, Northwestern University Feinberg School of Medicine, 303 E. Chicago Avenue, Chicago, IL 60611, U.S.A.

Abstract

Epithelial cells line virtually every organ cavity in the body and are important for vectorial transport through epithelial monolayers such as nutrient uptake or waste product excretion. Central to these tasks is the establishment of epithelial cell polarity. During organ development, epithelial cells set up two biochemically distinct plasma membrane domains, the apical and the basolateral domain. Targeting of correct constituents to each of these regions is essential for maintaining epithelial cell polarity. Newly synthesized transmembrane proteins destined for the basolateral or apical membrane domain are sorted into separate transport carriers either at the TGN (*trans*-Golgi network) or in perinuclear REs (recycling endosomes). After initial delivery, transmembrane proteins, such as nutrient receptors, frequently undergo multiple rounds of endocytosis followed by re-sorting in REs. Recent work in epithelial cells highlights the REs as a potent sorting station with different subdomains representing individual targeting zones that facilitate the correct surface delivery of transmembrane proteins.

[1]*To whom correspondence should be addressed (email h-folsch@northwestern.edu).*

Introduction

During polarization, epithelial cells segregate their plasma membrane into apical and basolateral domains, both enriched with a specific set of transmembrane proteins and lipids. For example, the apical membrane is enriched with glycolipids and cholesterol, whereas the basolateral membrane hosts cell adhesion proteins and nutrient receptors such as LDLR [LDL (low-density lipoprotein) receptor] and TfnR [Tfn (transferrin) receptor]. Apical and basolateral membranes are separated by tight junctions that serve as diffusion barriers. Furthermore, fully polarized simple epithelial cells, such as MDCK (Madin–Darby canine kidney) cells grow out a primary cilium from the apical membrane. The primary cilium represents a third distinct membrane domain with its own subset of constituents. Throughout the lifetime of individual epithelial cells it is important to faithfully sort transmembrane proteins and lipids to their correct target location to maintain polarity. Moreover, cells need to distinguish between proteins destined for plasma membrane domains or intracellular organelles, such as endosomes and lysosomes.

Transmembrane proteins destined for endosomes or lysosomes, or the different plasma membrane locations, typically move together from the endoplasmic reticulum to the Golgi apparatus. However, upon arrival at the TGN (*trans*-Golgi network), proteins are sorted away from each other by means of specific sorting signals encoded in either their luminal or transmembrane domains (majority of apical proteins), or cytoplasmic tails (majority of lysosomal and basolateral proteins), which are recognized by specialized sorting machineries. In general, cytoplasmic tail signals that direct a protein to the basolateral membrane are *cis*-dominant over apical sorting information. Moreover, not all proteins destined for the apical or basolateral domain are sorted at the TGN. Instead, some proteins move from the TGN into REs (recycling endosomes) for subsequent sorting.

Unlike REs in fibroblasts that do not have the specific task of sorting plasma membrane proteins to different membrane domains, REs in epithelial cells are much more elaborate, with domains involved in apical targeting [also named AREs (apical REs)] or basolateral targeting [also named CREs (common REs)] (reviewed in [1]). In fact, the sorting functions of both domains are so distinct that some groups believe they are entirely distinct REs (reviewed in [2]). Furthermore, it is highly likely that a third domain exists for trafficking into the primary cilium. In analogy to the model of Rab domains in EEs (early endosomes) established by Zerial and co-workers [3], the different RE domains may be established by Rab proteins involved in targeting processes. In addition to multi-faceted REs, epithelial cells also have two different kinds of EEs: AEEs (apical EEs) that underlie the apical membrane and BEEs (basolateral EEs) that underlie the basolateral membrane (reviewed in [1]). Proteins internalized from either membrane first arrive in AEEs or BEEs, from which they may immediately return to their membrane of origin or shuttle into REs for re-sorting.

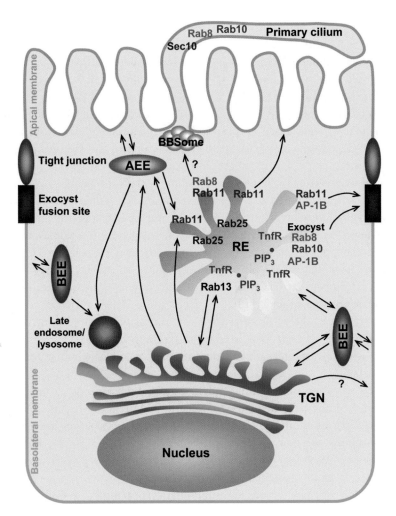

Figure 1. Model of different sorting pathways in a polarized epithelial cell
The sorting of biosynthetic cargos to different plasma membrane domains occurs either at the TGN or in the RE in a polarized epithelial cell. Arrows indicate the direction of movement of representative cargos at various compartments. Question marks denote pathways that are not yet proven. PIP_3, $PtdIns(3,4,5)P_3$.

In the following sections, surface delivery of transmembrane proteins will be discussed, with a focus on the endosomal compartments involved in these processes (summarized in Figure 1).

Sorting to the apical membrane

Cargos destined for the apical membrane have diverse sorting signals. The most common are perhaps N- or O-linked glycans attached to their luminal domains. These signals can be found in, for example, endolyn and the neurotrophin receptor p75. Other proteins, such as influenza HA (haemagglutinin), contain apical sorting information in their transmembrane domains. In addition, GPI (glycosylphosphatidylinositol) anchors may also serve as apical targeting determinants. Despite their diverse nature, a common theme is that apical targeting may be facilitated by sorting lectins of the galectin family that bind glycan residues at the luminal side of vesicles, thereby clustering the cargos for incorporation into transport carriers. Curiously, galectins are synthesized in the cytosol, and it is currently not clear how they end up in the lumen of nascent vesicles. In addition, apical cargos may also be clustered because of the physical properties of their sorting signals. Clustering of apical cargos occurs either into lipid raft or non-raft domains (reviewed in [4,5]).

Lipid rafts are defined as clusters of sphingolipids (glycosphingolipids and sphingomyelin) and cholesterol that are resistant to Triton X-100 extraction at 4°C (reviewed in [6]). Raft-dependent cargos, such as influenza HA and GPI-anchored proteins, are thought to associate with lipid rafts at the TGN. This association is mediated by a physical affinity to the raft lipids or may be facilitated by galectin-4 that has an affinity to glycosphingolipids. In addition, the PtdIns4P adaptor protein FAPP2 enhances apical delivery of raft-associated proteins (reviewed in [5]). Interestingly, instead of being directly delivered to the apical membrane, raft-associated cargos seem to travel to AEEs first where they mix with cargos internalized from the apical membrane before appearance on the surface [7].

Apical targeting of raft-independent cargos, such as endolyn or the neurotrophin receptor p75, depends on galectin-3. Furthermore, apical delivery of endolyn can be inhibited by ablating the apical sorting power of REs [7]. Proteins needed for apical targeting from REs are, for example, Rab11 and its effector myosin Vb [7]. Other apically targeted proteins, such as A-VSVG (apical variant of the vesicular stomatitis virus glycoprotein), were shown to move through recycling endosomal subdomains containing the TfnR (reviewed in [1]). Interestingly, TfnR-positive REs are thought to function as basolateral sorting stations. Most probably, A-VSVG moves together with proteins destined for the basolateral membrane from the TGN into REs, before segregating away into the apical pathway.

In conclusion, raft-dependent cargos seem to move through AEEs, whereas raft-independent cargos may move through Rab11-positive recycling endosomal domains, before arriving at the apical membrane.

Sorting to endosomes and the basolateral membrane

Sorting signals that direct proteins into the basolateral pathway are frequently encoded in the cytoplasmic tails of transmembrane proteins and consist of short dileucine (LL) or tyrosine-based (YxxØ or FxNPxY) peptide motifs. These signals are similar to endocytic motifs and lysosomal targeting determinants and are recognized by cytosolic adaptor complexes. There are monomeric clathrin adaptors like the TGN-localized GGA [Golgi-localized, γ-ear-containing, Arf

(ADP-ribosylation-factor)-binding] proteins and heterotetrameric AP (adaptor protein) complexes that may link cargo binding to the recruitment of clathrin. There are five main classes of heterotetrameric AP complexes, all of which have two large ~100 kDa subunits (γ, α, δ, ϵ, ζ and $\beta1$–$\beta5$), a medium ~50 kDa μ subunit, and a small ~20 kDa σ subunit. AP-2 facilitates clathrin-mediated endocytosis, AP-3 and AP-4 facilitate sorting of lysosomal cargos at the TGN or endosomes, and the AP-5 complex localizes to late endosomes [8,9]. In addition, epithelial cells express two highly homologous AP-1 complexes, AP-1A and the tissue-specific AP-1B. AP-1A and AP-1B share both large subunits and the small subunit, but differ in the incorporation of their respective medium subunit $\mu1A$ or $\mu1B$. Whereas AP-1A localizes at the TGN and endosomes and sorts proteins in the endosomal system, AP-1B exclusively localizes in TfnR-positive REs and is required for basolateral sorting from this location (reviewed in [1]). It is thought that $\mu1B$ empowers AP-1B with the necessary properties needed for basolateral sorting from REs. However, it is currently not entirely clear how this is possible given that $\mu1A$ and $\mu1B$ are ~80% identical at the amino acid level.

Sorting at the TGN

Interestingly, all AP complexes recognize similar sorting signals, yet they direct proteins into different targeting pathways towards endosomes and lysosomes, or towards the basolateral membrane. Perhaps subtle differences in the preferences for amino acid combinations in YxxØ motifs, where x describes any amino acid and Ø describes a hydrophobic residue, effect the efficiencies with which cargo is selected into nascent coated vesicles [10]. This would result in some proteins being preferentially incorporated into AP-1A, AP-3 or AP-4 vesicles at the TGN for sorting into the endosomal system. Moreover, some cargos with LL or YxxØ sorting signals are packaged at the TGN for basolateral surface delivery, and there has been some evidence that AP-4 may be involved in such a step (reviewed in [1]). An open question in the field is whether AP-1A and AP-3 may also participate in basolateral sorting. Furthermore, are there different coated vesicles leaving the TGN for endosomes and the basolateral membrane? Perhaps cargos packaged into coated vesicles at the TGN move together into BEEs, from which basolateral proteins reach their target membrane together with receptors that were internalized from that region. Indeed, low amounts of lysosomal transmembrane proteins such as lgp120 (120 kDa lysosomal membrane glycoprotein)/Lamp1 (lysosomal-associated membrane protein 1) are known to cycle through the basolateral membrane [11].

Sorting in REs

Some proteins with YxxØ motifs, such as VSVG, are not efficiently incorporated into transport vesicles at the TGN and travel instead into TfnR-positive REs. This step is regulated by Rab13 (reviewed in [1]). In REs, cargo may directly interact with AP-1B for basolateral sorting, or may interact with the co-adaptor ARH (autosomal recessive hypercholesterolaemia) protein. For example, LDLR encodes an FxNPxY sorting motif that is recognized by ARH in REs. ARH in turn interacts with AP-1B and thus facilitates AP-1B-dependent sorting of LDLR [12]. Notably, AP-1B is the only AP complex that localizes exclusively in REs. Membrane recruitment of AP-1B is facilitated by Arf6 and depends on PtdIns(3,4,5)P_3 [13,14]. Remarkably, PtdIns(3,4,5)P_3 is enriched in TfnR-positive REs, and depends on AP-1B expression. It is likely that PtdIns(3,4,5)P_3 is generated by a PIPKIγ-90 (PtdIns4P 5-kinase), in conjunction with a PI3K (phosphoinositide 3-kinase). PIPKIγ-90 directly interacts with AP-1B, and its localization in REs is dependent on AP-1B [13]. In REs, AP-1B triggers the recruitment of at least some subunits of the mammalian exocyst complex, Exo70 and Sec8, for incorporation into AP-1B vesicles. The exocyst is a vesicle-tethering complex thought to tie AP-1B vesicles to the basolateral membrane in a RalA-dependent manner. Additional regulators of the AP-1B pathway are Cdc42 (cell division cycle 42), Rab8 and Rab10 (reviewed in [1])

An interesting spin-off of AP-1B-dependent sorting through REs is the surface delivery of E-cadherin, which depends on PIPKIγ-90 and AP-1B. In addition, E-cadherin trafficking is dependent on Rab11 (reviewed in [1]). Thus E-cadherin may move through REs that contain markers of both basolateral and apical sorting domains.

In summary, basolateral cargos may be sorted at the TGN and subsequently may move through BEEs. Alternatively, basolateral cargos may move from the TGN into REs for sorting along the AP-1B pathway. Special features that μ1B bestows on AP-1B are an affinity for PtdIns(3,4,5)P_3 and the ability to trigger membrane recruitment of the exocyst complex, both features are needed for proper basolateral delivery from REs. The importance of AP-1B for epithelial cells is highlighted by the fact that proteins implicated in cancer development, such as EGFR [EGF (epidermal growth factor) receptor] and its ligand amphiregulin, depend on AP-1B for basolateral sorting [15,16], and researchers found that μ1B/AP-1B was down-regulated in colon cancer models and Crohn's disease patients [17,18]. This is especially interesting knowing that not all polarized epithelial cells express AP-1B, and AP-1B is, for example, not expressed in hepatocytes and cells derived from the renal proximal tubule (LLC-PK1 cells) [19].

Transcytosis

Some proteins are first delivered to the apical or basolateral membrane and after endocytosis are re-sorted to the opposite membrane domain in a process called apical-to-basolateral or basolateral-to-apical transcytosis. Common to both processes is that the internalized proteins need to reach REs for re-sorting. Perhaps one of the best-studied transcytotic proteins is pIgR [polymeric Ig (immunoglobulin) receptor] that mediates apical delivery of IgA. pIgR is first sorted to the basolateral membrane and can be found in BEEs and REs on its pathway (reviewed in [1]). Although the biosynthetic path of pIgR is not entirely clear, it has recently been suggested that at least its maintenance at the basolateral membrane depends on AP-1B [18]. After IgA binding, pIgR transcytoses from the basolateral membrane through TfnR-positive and Rab11-positive REs to the apical membrane [20]. Apical transcytosis depends on Rab11 and Rab25 [21]. Likewise, basolateral-to-apical transcytosis of NgCAM (neuron glia cell adhesion molecule) follows a path through Rab11-positive REs [22]. NgCAM has a YxxØ sorting motif in its cytoplasmic tail that is needed for basolateral recycling via AP-1B. This motif is phosphorylated during transcytosis, which inhibits AP-1B binding [23].

An interesting transcytotic receptor is FcRn that transports IgG across epithelial monolayers in both apical-to-basolateral and basolateral-to-apical directions. Transcytosis in both directions depends on Rab25 and myosin Vb. Curiously, Rab11 is necessary only for basolateral recycling [24]. Thus, besides E-cadherin, FcRn is the second known protein to require Rab11 for basolateral sorting.

Collectively, an emerging theme is that Rab25 regulates transcytosis in general. How exactly Rab25 works alongside Rab11 and other effectors of REs will be seen in the future.

Sorting into primary cilia

In recent years, investigation of sorting into primary cilia has gained much needed momentum. Central to this was the description of the so-called BBSome, an octameric complex of conserved Bardet–Biedl syndrome proteins that promotes ciliogenesis. The BBSome was described as a coat that forms on membranes, and *in vitro* work has suggested that the BBSome has highest affinity to PtdIns(3,4)P_2-positive membranes (reviewed in [25]). However, it is currently not clear where in the cell these membrane domains exist. Interestingly, INPP5E (inositol polyphosphate-5-phosphatase E) was linked to ciliopathies, such as Joubert syndrome. INPP5E hydrolyses the 5-phosphate of PtdIns(3,4,5)P_3 or PtdIns(4,5)P_2 [26]. This is interesting because, as discussed in the section on basolateral sorting, TfnR-positive REs are enriched in PtdIns(3,4,5)P_3. Perhaps membranes originating from REs play a role in targeting to cilia, and INPP5E is involved in creating a PtdIns(3,4)P_2-positive membrane domain from a PtdIns(3,4,5)P_3 pool.

In forming primary cilia, the BBSome co-operates with Rab8 (reviewed in [25]). In this process, Rab8 is activated via its exchange factor Rabin8, which in turn is activated by Rab11 [27]. Thus ciliogenesis involves Rab proteins that also work in the basolateral pathway (Rab8) or the apical pathway (Rab11). Although it is not clear at which intracellular compartment this activation cascade takes place, it is tempting to speculate that this may involve trafficking from a putative recycling endosomal subdomain where Rab8 and Rab11 may overlap. Intriguingly, other players already known for their role in basolateral sorting are also involved in ciliogenesis, such as the exocyst subunit Sec10 (reviewed in [28]), as well as Cdc42 [29] and perhaps Rab10. Although there are no data yet confirming a role for Rab10 in ciliogenesis, Rab10 antibodies were recently shown to stain the entire length of primary cilia [30].

Movement within the cilia is mediated by IFT (intraflagellar transport) particles. Interestingly, IFT88 levels are decreased upon knock down of Sec10. This indicates that the exocyst complex may regulate IFT88 transport into primary cilia, perhaps involving REs (reviewed in [28]). Ciliary delivery of other IFT proteins, such as IFT20, was shown to depend on the Golgi marker GMAP210 (Golgi microtubule-associated protein of 210 kDa)/TRIP11 (thyroid receptor-interacting protein 11) (reviewed in [25]). This suggests that transport of IFT20 to the cilia perhaps follows a direct pathway from the Golgi.

Taken together, the outgrowth of primary cilia involves protein complexes specific for cilia (BBSome, IFT proteins), and components that this pathway shares with apical (Rab11) or basolateral (Rab8, Cdc42 and Sec10) pathways. Furthermore, components may reach cilia directly from the Golgi or perhaps from REs. However, despite these clear advances, many issues concerning the molecular mechanisms of ciliogenesis remain unresolved.

Conclusions

Apical or basolateral proteins were once thought to be packaged into different transport carriers at the TGN during biosynthetic delivery followed by direct transport, without traversing endosomes, to their target membrane. REs were then thought to 'just' sort internalized cargos, and they came in two flavours: Rab11-positive REs for apical targeting and TfnR-positive REs for basolateral targeting. Both viewpoints have been challenged in recent years. First, through ablation of endosomal compartments, researchers find ever more evidence which indicates that instead of being sorted directly from the TGN to the plasma membrane, cargos move through endosomes to reach their final destination. However, more work is needed to fully understand the role of endosomes in biosynthetic targeting. Secondly, we can no longer look at REs as a compartment with just two simple specifications. Instead, recent advances indicate that REs possess a high plasticity to accommodate the specific sorting needs of a diverse range of transmembrane proteins. Still, it is currently not entirely clear how different subdomains of REs are formed, perhaps with the help of Rab proteins. Notably, in biosynthetic surface delivery REs emerge as a post-TGN compartment with perhaps equal sorting capacity to the TGN, and it is in REs that internalized proteins are correctly delivered back to the plasma membrane. This is a rapidly evolving field and it is increasingly becoming clear that the correct sorting of proteins implicated in, for example, cancer development is important for disease prevention.

Note added in proof

During the production of the present chapter, a study was published that showed a role for AP-1A in sorting of basolateral proteins at the TGN [31]. That study fits very well with the model we present in the current chapter.

Summary

- *Epithelial cells distinguish at least three different plasma membrane locations: apical domain, basolateral domain and primary cilia.*
- *Plasma membrane proteins encode targeting signals in their luminal domains or cytoplasmic tails that are recognized by specific sorting machineries.*
- *Biosynthetic delivery of transmembrane proteins to the plasma membrane frequently involves the passage through endosomes.*
- *Basolateral and lysosomal proteins encode similar sorting signals in their cytoplasmic tails that are recognized by cytosolic AP complexes, and lysosomal proteins cycle exclusively through the basolateral membrane.*
- *REs present a plastic sorting station with multiple subdomains that aid in correct protein sorting of endocytic and biosynthetic cargos.*
- *AP-1B is instrumental in basolateral sorting from REs where it facilitates the generation of its own recycling endosomal subdomain.*
- *Primary cilia emerge from the apical membrane when epithelial cells are fully polarized. Ciliogenesis requires some proteins that are also involved in apical or basolateral targeting, highlighting the plasticity of sorting pathways.*

We apologize to all researchers whose work we were unable to include because of space limitations. This work was supported by the National Institutes of Health [grant number GM070736] to H.F. S.F.A was supported by an A*STAR Singapore postdoctoral fellowship.

References

1. Fölsch, H., Mattila, P.E. and Weisz, O.A. (2009) Taking the scenic route: biosynthetic traffic to the plasma membrane in polarized epithelial cells. Traffic **10**, 972–981
2. Mostov, K., Su, T. and ter Beest, M. (2003) Polarized epithelial membrane traffic: conservation and plasticity. Nat. Cell Biol. **5**, 287–293
3. Rink, J., Ghigo, E., Kalaidzidis, Y. and Zerial, M. (2005) Rab conversion as a mechanism of progression from early to late endosomes. Cell **122**, 735–749
4. Weisz, O.A. and Rodriguez-Boulan, E (2009) Apical trafficking in epithelial cells: signals, clusters and motors. J. Cell Sci. **122**, 4253–4266
5. Fölsch, H (2008) Regulation of membrane trafficking in polarized epithelial cells. Curr. Opin. Cell Biol. **20**, 208–213
6. Schuck, S. and Simons, K. (2004) Polarized sorting in epithelial cells: raft clustering and the biogenesis of the apical membrane. J. Cell Sci. **117**, 5955–5964
7. Cresawn, K.O., Potter, B.A., Oztan, A., Guerriero, C.J., Ihrke, G., Goldenring, J.R., Apodaca, G. and Weisz, O.A. (2007) Differential involvement of endocytic compartments in the biosynthetic traffic of apical proteins. EMBO J **26**, 3737–3748
8. Boehm, M. and Bonifacino, J.S. (2001) Adaptins: the final recount. Mol. Biol. Cell **12**, 2907–2920
9. Hirst, J., Barlow, L.D., Francisco, G.C., Sahlender, D.A., Seaman, M.N., Dacks, J.B. and Robinson, M.S. (2011) The fifth adaptor protein complex. PLoS Biol. **9**, e1001170

10. Ohno, H., Fournier, M.C., Poy, G. and Bonifacino, J.S. (1996) Structural determinants of interaction of tyrosine-based sorting signals with the adaptor medium chains. J. Biol. Chem. **271**, 29009–29015

11. Hunziker, W., Harter, C., Matter, K. and Mellman, I. (1991) Basolateral sorting in MDCK cells requires a distinct cytoplasmic domain determinant. Cell **66**, 907–920

12. Kang, R.S. and Fölsch, H. (2011) ARH cooperates with AP-1B in the exocytosis of LDLR in polarized epithelial cells. J. Cell Biol. **193**, 51–60

13. Fields, I.C., King, S.M., Shteyn, E., Kang, R.S. and Fölsch, H. (2010) Phosphatidylinositol 3,4,5-trisphosphate localization in recycling endosomes is necessary for AP-1B-dependent sorting in polarized epithelial cells. Mol. Biol. Cell **21**, 95–105

14. Shteyn, E., Pigati, L. and Fölsch, H. (2011) Arf6 regulates AP-1B-dependent sorting in polarized epithelial cells. J. Cell Biol. **194**, 873–887

15. Gephart, J.D., Singh, B., Higginbotham, J.N., Franklin, J.L., Gonzalez, A., Fölsch, H. and Coffey, R.J. (2011) Identification of a novel mono-leucine basolateral sorting motif within the cytoplasmic domain of amphiregulin. Traffic **12**, 1793–1804

16. Ryan, S., Verghese, S., Cianciola, N.L., Cotton, C.U. and Carlin, C.R. (2010) Autosomal recessive polycystic kidney disease epithelial cell model reveals multiple basolateral epidermal growth factor receptor sorting pathways. Mol. Biol. Cell 2010, **21**, 2732–2745

17. Mimura, M., Masuda, A., Nishiumi, S., Kawakami, K., Fujishima, Y., Yoshie, T., Mizuno, S., Miki, I., Ohno, H., Hase, K. et al. (2012) AP1B plays an important role in intestinal tumorigenesis with the truncating mutation of an APC gene. Int. J. Cancer **130**, 1011–1020

18. Takahashi, D., Hase, K., Kimura, S., Nakatsu, F., Ohmae, M., Mandai, Y., Sato, T., Date, Y., Ebisawa, M., Kato, T. et al. (2011) The epithelia-specific membrane trafficking factor AP-1B controls gut immune homeostasis in mice. Gastroenterology **141**, 621–632

19. Ohno, H., Tomemori, T., Nakatsu, F., Okazaki, Y., Aguilar, R.C., Fölsch, H., Mellman, I., Saito, T., Shirasawa, T. and Bonifacino, J.S. (1999) Mu1B, a novel adaptor medium chain expressed in polarized epithelial cells. FEBS Lett. **449**, 215–220

20. Su, T., Bryant, D.M., Luton, F., Verges, M., Ulrich, S.M., Hansen, K.C., Datta, A., Eastburn, D.J., Burlingame, A.L., Shokat, K.M. et al. (2010) A kinase cascade leading to Rab11-FIP5 controls transcytosis of the polymeric immunoglobulin receptor. Nat. Cell Biol. **12**, 1143–1153

21. Wang, X., Kumar, R., Navarre, J., Casanova, J.E. and Goldenring, J.R. (2000) Regulation of vesicle trafficking in Madin–Darby canine kidney cells by Rab11a and Rab25. J. Biol. Chem. **275**, 29138–29146

22. Thompson, A., Nessler, R., Wisco, D., Anderson, E., Winckler, B. and Sheff, D. (2007) Recycling endosomes of polarized epithelial cells actively sort apical and basolateral cargos into separate subdomains. Mol. Biol. Cell **18**, 2687–2697

23. Anderson, E., Maday, S., Sfakianos, J., Hull, M., Winckler, B., Sheff, D., Fölsch, H. and Mellman, I. (2005) Transcytosis of NgCAM in epithelial cells reflects differential signal recognition on the endocytic and secretory pathways. J. Cell Biol. **170**, 595–605

24. Tzaban, S., Massol, R.H., Yen, E., Hamman, W., Frank, S.R., Lapierre, L.A., Hansen, S.H., Goldenring, J.R., Blumberg, R.S. and Lencer, W.I. (2009) The recycling and transcytotic pathways for IgG transport by FcRn are distinct and display an inherent polarity. J. Cell Biol. **185**, 673–684

25. Nachury, M.V., Seeley, E.S. and Jin, H. (2010) Trafficking to the ciliary membrane: how to get across the periciliary diffusion barrier? Annu. Rev. Cell Dev. Biol. **26**, 59–87

26. Bielas, S.L., Silhavy, J.L., Brancati, F., Kisseleva, M.V., Al-Gazali, L., Sztriha, L., Bayoumi, R.A., Zaki, M.S., Abdel-Aleem, A., Rosti, R.O. et al. (2009) Mutations in INPP5E, encoding inositol polyphosphate-5-phosphatase E, link phosphatidyl inositol signaling to the ciliopathies. Nat. Genet. **41**, 1032–1036

27. Knodler, A., Feng, S., Zhang, J., Zhang, X., Das, A., Peranen, J. and Guo, W. (2010) Coordination of Rab8 and Rab11 in primary ciliogenesis. Proc. Natl. Acad. Sci. U.S.A. **107**, 6346–6351

28. Kang, R.S. and Folsch, H. (2009) An old dog learns new tricks: novel functions of the exocyst complex in polarized epithelia in animals. F1000 Biol. Rep. **1**, 83

29. Zuo, X., Fogelgren, B. and Lipschutz, J.H. (2011) The small GTPase Cdc42 is necessary for primary ciliogenesis in renal tubular epithelial cells. J. Biol. Chem. **286**, 22469–22477

30. Babbey, C.M., Bacallao, R.L. and Dunn, K.W. (2010) Rab10 associates with primary cilia and the exocyst complex in renal epithelial cells. Am. J. Physiol. Renal Physiol. **299**, F495–F506

31. Gravotta, D., Carvajal-Gonzalez, J.M., Mattera, R., Deborde, S., Banfelder, J.R., Bonifacino, J.S. and Rodriguez-Boulan, E. (2012) The clathrin adaptor AP-1A mediates basolateral polarity. Dev. Cell **22**, 811–823

© The Authors Journal compilation © 2012 Biochemical Society
Essays Biochem. (2012) 53, 41–54: doi: 10.1042/BSE0530041

4

Continuous endocytic recycling of tight junction proteins: how and why?

Andrew D. Chalmers and Paul Whitley

Department of Biology and Biochemistry, Centre for Regenerative Medicine, University of Bath, Bath BA2 7AY, U.K.

Abstract

Tight junctions consist of many proteins, including transmembrane and associated cytoplasmic proteins, which act to provide a barrier regulating transport across epithelial and endothelial tissues. These junctions are dynamic structures that are able to maintain barrier function during tissue remodelling and rapidly alter it in response to extracellular signals. Individual components of tight junctions also show dynamic behaviour, including migration within the junction and exchange in and out of the junctions. In addition, it is becoming clear that some tight junction proteins undergo continuous endocytosis and recycling back to the plasma membrane. Regulation of endocytic trafficking of junctional proteins may provide a way of rapidly remodelling junctions and will be the focus of this chapter.

An introduction to tight junctions

Tight junctions were first identified in electron micrographs, which revealed close contacts linking adjacent epithelial cells [1]. These junctions, which are also found in endothelial cells, provide a barrier that regulates diffusion through

Correspondence may be addressed to either author (email ac270@bath.ac.uk or bssprw@bath.ac.uk).

the paracellular space (Figure 1). The history, function and molecular compo-nents of the tight junctions has been reviewed recently [2,3]. In the present chapter we will provide a brief introduction to tight junctions before focusing on their dynamic nature, and in particular the endocytic recycling of individual tight junction proteins.

Although tight junctions provide a barrier to diffusion, this barrier is not absolute as it allows the passage of certain solutes [2]. In addition the permeabil-ity of tight junctions varies between different epithelial cells so that some epi-thelia form a 'tight' barrier whereas others are 'leaky'. Tight junctions not only provide a barrier, but there is growing evidence they act as a platform for cell signalling molecules that regulate cellular behaviours, including gene expression and cell proliferation rates [4].

Molecular studies have shown that tight junctions consist of a large number of proteins, including members of the claudin, occludin and JAM (junctional adhesion molecule) families of transmembrane proteins [2]. The claudin pro-teins, consisting of over 20 members in humans, are thought to be the main mediators of the epithelial permeability barrier [5–7]. There are many lines of evidence to support this hypothesis, for example claudins can promote tight junction strand formation when expressed in fibroblasts [8] and mouse knock-out studies show alterations in barrier function in a wide range of tissues,

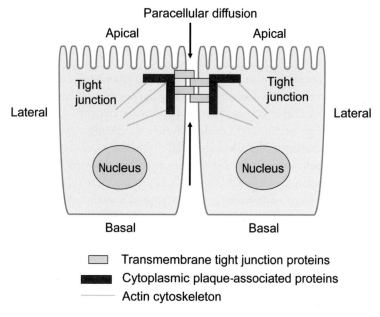

Figure 1. Tight junctions provide a barrier that regulates paracellular diffusion across epithelial sheets
Tight junctions consist of many proteins including transmembrane proteins of the occludin, clau-din and JAM families and associated cytoplasmic proteins including ZO-1 and cingulin. The trans-membrane proteins are thought to mediate the permeability barrier, whereas the adaptor proteins link the junctions to the cytoskeleton and recruit cell signalling proteins.

including the skin for claudin-1 knockouts [9] and kidney for claudin-2 knockouts [10]. Importantly, some claudins promote a high-resistance barrier to diffusion, whereas others are thought to form pores that allow ionic diffusion [5]. Thus variations in the expression profile of claudins is proposed to be a major determinant of tissue-specific variations in permeability [7]. The other transmembrane tight junction proteins appear to have a role in the regulation/modulation of this claudin-based barrier [2,3]. A range of cytoplasmic proteins can associate with the transmembrane proteins, such as ZO (zonula occludens)-1 and cingulin, which indirectly link tight junctions to the actin cytoskeleton and various signalling proteins [11–13]. The formation of these large multi-subunit structures allows the tight junctions to fulfil the various functions associated with them, including barrier formation and regulation of cell signalling.

The dynamic nature of tight junctions

Tight junctions are found in tissues that show dynamic behaviours. For example, in the mammalian intestine, epithelial cells are replaced every 4–5 days [14], and during pregnancy there is a massive increase in mammary epithelial cells which are then removed at the end of lactation [15]. During the addition and removal of cells, tight junctions must be able to maintain barrier function. Tight junctions must also be remodelled as immune cells transmigrate through epithelia and during wound healing [3]. Many stimuli, including inflammatory cytokines and bacterial infection, also rapidly modify the tight junction barrier [16]. These observations suggest that rapid alteration of tight junction composition occurs and there is general acceptance that tight junctions, like the epithelial tissues they are found in, are dynamic structures. The dynamic behaviour of the tight junctions includes movement of tight junction strands and of individual tight junction proteins, which can diffuse within the tight junctions and in and out of the junctions [2,3]. There also appears to be continuous endocytosis and recycling back to the plasma membrane of tight junction proteins in a range of epithelial cell types [17–19], an aspect of tight junction dynamics that will be the focus of the present chapter.

Is continuous recycling of tight junction proteins a common feature of epithelial cells?

Following endocytosis from the plasma membrane into EEs (early endosomes), transmembrane cargo proteins can follow the degradative pathway to the lysosome or be recycled back to the plasma membrane. They can also undergo retrograde transport to the TGN (*trans*-Golgi network) where they may undergo further sorting [20]. In epithelial cells the picture is further complicated by endocytosis from distinct apical and basolateral membrane domains into apical or basolateral EEs and transcytosis between the two domains [4,21] (Figure 2). There are also multiple independent pathways responsible for recycling

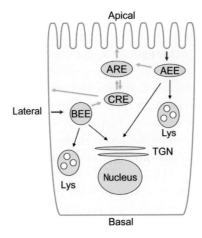

Figure 2. Endocytic trafficking routes in a polarized epithelial cell
Schematic diagram providing an overview of endocytic trafficking routes in epithelial cells; however, characterization of these routes is ongoing and endocytic trafficking is likely to be more complicated than presented here. There are also likely to be cell-type-specific and stimuli-induced variations in trafficking. AEE, apical EE; ARE, apical RE; BEE, basal EE; CRE, common recycling endosome; LYS, lysosome.

proteins back to the plasma membrane [22] making endocytic protein trafficking, particularly in epithelial cells, an extremely complex process.

Identifying the trafficking fate of an endocytosed transmembrane tight junction protein can be achieved using a biotinylation assay that labels extracellular lysine residues of proteins allowing their trafficking to be monitored [23]. The biotinylation assay was used to provide the first evidence that tight junction proteins can be continuously recycled in confluent epithelial cells when occludin was found to be endocytosed and recycled back to the plasma membrane in a mouse mammary cell line (MTD1A) [19]. In contrast, claudin-1 was not endocytosed in these cells. However, a potential limitation of this study is that the rate of degradation of occludin was not measured. Owing to the nature of the biotinylation assay used it is possible that at least some of the occludin trafficking classified as recycling could have been a consequence of degradation.

Subsequent experiments with MDCK (Madin–Darby canine kidney) II cells, a canine kidney line [17] which is commonly used to study tight junctions, examined the trafficking of claudin-1 and occludin. Importantly, this work added an additional control so that degradation and recycling could be distinguished. Claudin-1 was found to be constantly endocytosed and recycled in MDCK II cells, with no detectable degradation observed over the time frame of these assays (20 min for degradation and recycling). Over longer time periods (hours/days) claudin-1 is degraded [24], indicating that a small percentage of endocytosed claudin-1 is directed for degradation in MDCK II cells. This would produce a gradual turnover of claudin-1 protein. Subsequent work showed that, like claudin-1, claudin-2 is endocytosed and recycled in MDCK II cells [18]. In contrast, significant endocytosis of occludin [17] and claudin-4 [18]

Table 1. Continuous recycling of tight junction proteins in polarized epithelial monolayers

The continuous recycling of tight junction proteins has been studied in the canine kidney line MDCK II, the human colon cancer line CaCo-2, the human lung epithelial line 16-HBE and the mouse mammary line MTD-1A.

Tight junction proteins	MDCK II	CaCo-2	16-HBE	MTD-1A
Claudin-1	Recycled [17]	Recycled [17]	Recycled [17]	Not endocytosed* [19]
Claudin-2	Recycled [18]	–	–	–
Claudin-4	Not endocytosed* [18]	–	–	–
Occludin	Not endocytosed* [17]	Degraded and recycled [17]	Degraded and recycled [17]	Recycled [19]

*There was no detectable endocytosis in the time frame of the biotinylation assays (often 1 h), but there may be a lower rate of endocytosis which would produce a gradual turnover in protein.

was not detected in MDCK II cells using the same assay and incubation time (1 h), showing that tight junction proteins have different rates of flux through the endocytic system.

Analysis of additional epithelial cell lines showed that claudin-1 is constantly recycled in the human colon-cancer-derived line CaCo-2 and the human-lung-derived line 16-HBE [17]. Interestingly, unlike in MDCK II cells, in these lines occludin was endocytosed. Its fate was then split, with some protein being recycled and the rest being degraded. Combining results from the four different epithelial cell lines currently analysed shows that recycling of at least a subset of tight junction proteins is a common feature of epithelial cells. In addition there is cell-type-specific variation in the rate at which individual tight junction proteins are trafficked through the endocytic system. This data is summarized in Table 1. Most of this work is very recent and there are a number of issues that remain to be addressed. For example, it will be important to determine which other tight junction proteins are recycled and whether similar rates of recycling occur *in vivo*. It is also important to stress that the biotin assay does not label cytoplasmic proteins. This means it cannot be used to follow the fate of proteins such as ZO-1, which could be transported with the transmembrane tight junction proteins they associate with.

How is endocytosis of tight junction proteins mediated?

The first step in endocytic trafficking is the internalization of transmembrane proteins from the plasma membrane. Endocytosis can occur via clathrin-dependent [25] and clathrin-independent mechanisms, which include caveolae-driven endocytosis and macropinocytosis [26]. Endocytosis of tight junction proteins has been reported to occur by all of these mechanisms: for example calcium depletion, a non-physiological stimulus that induces tight junction breakdown, triggers endocytosis of occludin, claudin-1 and JAM-A by a clathrin-mediated pathway [27]. Studies on stimulus-induced remodelling have revealed clathrin-independent internalization of tight junction proteins. For example, occludin endocytosis occurs via caveolae following *Escherichia coli* CNF-1 (cytotoxic necrotizing factor-1) stimulation [28] or TNFα (tumour necrosis factor α) stimulation [16]. Recent work also shows that the chloride channel CIC-2 acts to reduce caveolae-mediated endocytosis of occludin in CaCo-2 cells [29]. Claudin-1, occludin and JAM-A are internalized via macropinocytosis in IFNγ (interferon γ)-treated T84 cells [30]. Live imaging studies using fluorescent fusion proteins have revealed a further feature of endocytosis for claudin-3 [31]. This involves a peculiar mechanism whereby plasma membranes from two juxtaposed cells are internalized into one of the cells. This has been referred to as 'eat-each-other' endocytosis.

It should also be noted that different tight junction proteins are not always endocytosed en masse, but can be endocytosed independently of one another. For example, EGF (epidermal growth factor) stimulation of MDCK II cells increases endocytosis and degradation of claudin-2 without affecting claudin-1 [32]. In addition, occludin endocytosis occurs in latrunculin-A-treated MDCK II cells [33] and *in vivo* in anti-CD3-treated mice [34] without concomitant internalization of claudin proteins. The ability to independently endocytose proteins may allow cells to alter the repertoire of tight junction proteins at the plasma membrane and fine-tune paracellular permeability in response to changing conditions.

An interesting question is what determines the selection of tight junction proteins as endocytic cargo, and one possibility is that post-translational modification of individual tight junction proteins is responsible. Ubiquitination, phosphorylation and palmitoylation are reversible modifications that have all been linked to endocytosis [21]. Transmembrane tight junction proteins have also been shown to undergo these modifications [35,36]. Expression of the ubiquitin ligase LNX1p80 drives endocytosis of claudin-1 [24], whereas an alternative ubiquitin ligase Itch promotes endocytosis of occludin [37]. An attractive hypothesis is that low level activity of these, and possibly other ubiquitin ligases, promotes continuous endocytosis of tight junction proteins. Regulation of specific ubiquitin ligase activity could also alter endocytic rates of individual tight junction components. However, knockdown or knockout experiments ablating the function of these proteins and analysis of the effect on endocytosis rates are required to establish if this is the case. Phosphorylation of claudins, occludin and JAMs have all been reported, with the phosphorylation status having an affect on tight junction localization [38–41]. For example, phosphorylation of Ser[490] of occludin is associated with its endocytosis and barrier loss in endothelial cells [42]. Finally, claudin family proteins contain conserved signature cysteine residues that are palmitoylated and are required for efficient localization at tight junctions [43]. Palmitoylation is a reversible protein modification that has been linked to endocytosis [44] in addition to other protein trafficking events [21,45,46] making it a potential regulator of claudin endocytosis.

Another important issue is where endocytosis of tight junction proteins occurs. It is plausible that tight junction proteins are not endocytosed from the junctions themselves, but from adjacent (or even distant) regions of the plasma membrane. Live imaging and computer modelling experiments have been performed to investigate the dynamics of individual tight junction components in living cells [47]. These studies indicate that occludin within the tight junctions continuously exchanges with an extra-tight junction pool. Furthermore, claudin-1 is located in the lateral membrane in addition to the junctional complexes of polarized epithelial cells [48–50]. Cytoskeletal rearrangements at tight junctions are likely to be crucial in facilitating junctional remodelling and endocytosis. If endocytosis occurs away from the tight junctions, then regulation of the rate that tight junction proteins move out of junctions and into regions of the plasma membrane undergoing active endocytosis would provide another possible mechanism of regulating endocytic cargo selection. The mechanisms, pathways and modifications mentioned are not mutually exclusive, and a complex interplay is likely to regulate selection for endocytosis.

Regulation of recycling and junctional remodelling

While many studies have considered stimulated endocytosis as an important process in tight junction remodelling, relatively little attention has focussed on post-endocytic sorting of tight junction components. However, the continuous recycling of junctional proteins [17–19] raises the possibility that a reduction in the rate of recycling could achieve the same goal as increased endocytosis, that is, removing tight junction proteins from the plasma membrane and causing either an accumulation of internal protein or increased degradation. The post-translational modifications, ubiquitination, phosphorylation and palmitoylation, mentioned above, all have roles to play in post-endocytic sorting [21], in addition to endocytosis, and so provide potential signals to regulate the rate of recycling of tight junction components. This leads to the question of whether control of post-endocytic sorting, in particular recycling, participates in junctional remodelling.

Evidence to suggest that control of post-endocytic sorting is important comes from studies on the fate of tight junction proteins in IFNγ-treated epithelial cells [30,51]. Occludin, claudin-1 and JAM-A all accumulate intracellularly, in compartments containing RE (recycling endosome) markers Rab4 and Rab11, following IFNγ treatment, with no increase in degradation of these proteins. Removal of IFNγ results in release of the accumulated proteins back to tight junctions, so it is reasonable to postulate that IFNγ treatment blocks recycling. Similarly, other manipulations of epithelial cells, such as removal of calcium [27] or incubation with CNF-1 [28], reversibly displace tight junction proteins to intracellular locations, indicating that regulation of recycling may be a common mechanism by which tight junction composition can be controlled. Intriguingly, following CNF-1 treatment, occludin does not co-localize intracellularly with claudin or JAM-A, providing evidence that these proteins could be recycled by distinct routes. Control of tight junction recycling is not limited to epithelial cells as claudin-5 and occludin recycle in endothelial cells following recovery from chemokine treatment [52].

Post-endocytic sorting and trafficking of tight junction proteins

In order to understand how stimuli might modify post-endocytic trafficking it is important to establish the endocytic routes taken by tight junction proteins and identify the proteins responsible for this trafficking. Following endocytosis the EEs are the primary destination for material removed from the plasma membrane. Proteins entering these endosomes must be sorted to degradative, recycling or retrograde endocytic trafficking pathways and this sorting is a major determinant of the fate of endocytosed proteins [21].

A group of proteins which are tightly linked to post-endocytic sorting is the ESCRT (endosomal sorting complex required for transport). This complex has a well-established role in the trafficking of ubiquitinated transmembrane proteins to lysosomes for degradation [53,54] and is important for attenuating signalling from growth factor receptors such as the EGFR (EGF receptor) [55]. However, in addition to blocking the degradative pathway, inhibiting ESCRT function can cause defects in the recycling of receptors, such as those for EGF, transferrin, asialoglycoprotein and low-density lipoprotein [56–59]. Experiments using a dominant-negative ESCRT protein showed that ESCRT function is required for the continuous recycling of claudin-1, and when ESCRT function is inhibited claudin-1 accumulates intracellularly [17]. Why is ESCRT function required for claudin-1 recycling? ESCRT proteins are known to interact with deubiquitinating enzymes, and the timing of deubiquitination is emerging as an important factor in modulating the fate of endocytosed proteins [60,61]. Therefore it is possible that perturbations in the ESCRT machinery leads to mis-regulation of ESCRT-associated deubiquitinating enzymes resulting in incorrect post-endocytic sorting and a failure in claudin-1 recycling.

Addition of YM201636, a small molecule inhibitor of the lipid kinase PIKfyve (FYVE finger-containing phosphoinositide kinase) also inhibits claudin-1 and claudin-2 recycling [18]. This kinase is responsible for the synthesis of $PtdIns(3,5)P_2$ from $PtdIns3P$ on early endosomes and its function has been linked to a number of endocytic sorting events [62,63]. It is unclear why PIKfyve function might be required for recycling of claudins, but as $PtdIns(3,5)$ P_2 binds the ESCRT III component Vps24 (vacuolar protein sorting 24)/ CHMP3 *in vitro* [64], it is possible that recycling is blocked by inhibiting the recruitment of the ESCRT machinery to endosomes.

Members of the Rab family of small GTPases have well-documented roles in vesicular trafficking [65], and experiments using a dominant-negative construct showed that Rab13 is required for the continuous recycling of occludin in MTD1A cells [19]. siRNA (small interfering RNA) knockdown experiments have also shown that the trafficking of internalized claudin-1 to the plasma membrane after a calcium switch (calcium depletion and subsequent repletion) requires Rab13 and its binding protein JRAB/MICAL-L2 [66]. This identifies Rab13 as a key mediator of tight junction recycling, although it also has an additional role in the biosynthetic delivery of cargoes from the TGN to endosomes in polarized epithelial cells [67]. Rab11 is well known to be involved in recycling, and tight junction proteins accumulate in Rab11-positive compartments following stimulation with IFNγ or CNF-1 [28,30], but we are not aware of any studies that have investigated the requirement of Rab11 in tight junction protein recycling. The ESCRT, PIKfyve and Rab13 studies described above have identified the first few proteins whose function is required for continuous tight junction recycling. However, it is clear that much more research is needed to provide a full description of the molecular basis for these events and to elucidate how specificity of recycling of individual tight junction proteins is achieved.

Why do cells continuously recycle tight junction proteins?

The final, and perhaps most important, question is why should cells expend the energy required to constantly move tight junction proteins into the cell and then back to the cell surface? A simple explanation is that no system is perfect and as some proteins may be internalized inappropriately, recycling would provide an efficient system to return these to the plasma membrane. Tight junction recycling may also have evolved as a consequence of the dynamic nature of tight junctions. If a cell needs to form more tight junctions it can reduce endocytosis and/or increase the rate of recycling to increase the amount of tight junctions at the cell surface. Conversely, if the area of tight junctions needs decreasing a cell can promote endocytosis and/or reduce recycling to remove excess tight junction proteins from the plasma membrane. This provides a flexible way to rapidly deal with physiological variations in tight junction size. It could also be used to fine-tune barrier function: for example, the composition of claudins at the plasma membrane could be altered to allow cells/tissues to regulate paracellular permeability.

The recycling of tight junctions may also be important in pathological conditions. Alterations of tight junctions have been associated with tumour formation [68] and blocking recycling would reduce the amount of functional tight junction protein at the plasma membrane, perhaps reducing the stability of epithelial tissues. Modulation of tight junctions also occurs in inflammatory bowel disease and following bacterial infection [16,28,30,51]. The evidence described above suggests that inflammatory cytokines and bacterial proteins may act, in part, by blocking tight junction recycling. These potential links to disease illustrate the importance of future work aimed at fully understanding this process.

Conclusions

The demonstration that tight junction recycling appears to be a common feature of epithelial cells throws up many questions such as how is it controlled and why is it important? Our understanding is still at a rudimentary level: tight junction recycling is known to occur in several different types of epithelial cells and the first few proteins which are required for this process have been identified, but many more experiments are required to provide a true mechanistic understanding. Key issues that need to be addressed include (i) what proteins mediate trafficking through the endocytic system, (ii) is there more than one tight junction recycling pathway and (iii) whether this process is regulated. Rates of recycling *in vivo* also need to be determined and, finally, the question of whether tight junction recycling is altered during pathological conditions such as cancer, inflammatory bowel diseases and bacterial infection needs to be addressed.

Summary

- *Tight junctions provide a permeability barrier that is dynamic and constantly undergoing remodelling.*
- *A number of tight junction components, including claudins and occludin, are constitutively endocytosed and recycled in epithelial cells.*
- *There is cell-type-specific variation in the tight junction proteins that are recycled.*
- *ESCRT, PIKfyve and Rab13 are required for tight junction recycling.*
- *Tight junction recycling may be aberrantly regulated in disease.*

Work in our laboratory on this area was supported by a Cancer Research UK project grant [grant number C26932/A9548]. We thank Dr Christopher Caunt (University of Bath) for critical comments on the draft of the chapter.

References

1. Farquhar, M.G. and Palade, G.E. (1963) Junctional complexes in various epithelia. J. Cell Biol. **17**, 375–412
2. Shen, L., Weber, C.R., Raleigh, D.R., Yu, D. and Turner, J.R. (2011) Tight junction pore and leak pathways: a dynamic duo. Annu. Rev. Physiol. **73**, 283–309
3. Steed, E., Balda, M.S. and Matter, K. (2010) Dynamics and functions of tight junctions. Trends Cell Biol. **20**, 142–149

4. Spadaro, D., Tapia, R., Pulimeno, P. and Citi, S. (2012) The control of gene expression and cell proliferation by the epithelial apical junctional complex. Essays Biochem. **53**, 83–93

5. Koval, M. (2006) Claudins: key pieces in the tight junction puzzle. Cell Commun. Adhes. **13**, 127–138

6. Krause, G., Winkler, L., Mueller, S.L., Haseloff, R.F., Piontek, J. and Blasig, I.E. (2008) Structure and function of claudins. Biochim. Biophys. Acta **1778**, 631–645

7. Van Itallie, C.M. and Anderson, J.M. (2006) Claudins and epithelial paracellular transport. Annu. Rev. Physiol. **68**, 403–429

8. Furuse, M., Sasaki, H., Fujimoto, K. and Tsukita, S. (1998) A single gene product, claudin-1 or -2, reconstitutes tight junction strands and recruits occludin in fibroblasts. J. Cell Biol. **143**, 391–401

9. Furuse, M., Hata, M., Furuse, K., Yoshida, Y., Haratake, A., Sugitani, Y., Noda, T., Kubo, A. and Tsukita, S. (2002) Claudin-based tight junctions are crucial for the mammalian epidermal barrier: a lesson from claudin-1-deficient mice. J. Cell Biol. **156**, 1099–1111

10. Muto, S., Hata, M., Taniguchi, J., Tsuruoka, S., Moriwaki, K., Saitou, M., Furuse, K., Sasaki, H., Fujimura, A., Imai, M. et al. (2010) Claudin-2-deficient mice are defective in the leaky and cation-selective paracellular permeability properties of renal proximal tubules. Proc. Natl. Acad. Sci. U.S.A. **107**, 8011–8016

11. Cordenonsi, M., D'Atri, F., Hammar, E., Parry, D.A., Kendrick-Jones, J., Shore, D. and Citi, S. (1999) Cingulin contains globular and coiled-coil domains and interacts with ZO-1, ZO-2, ZO-3, and myosin. J. Cell Biol. **147**, 1569–1582

12. D'Atri, F. and Citi, S. (2001) Cingulin interacts with F-actin *in vitro*. FEBS Lett. **507**, 21–24

13. Fanning, A.S., Jameson, B.J., Jesaitis, L.A. and Anderson, J.M. (1998) The tight junction protein ZO-1 establishes a link between the transmembrane protein occludin and the actin cytoskeleton. J. Biol. Chem. **273**, 29745–29753

14. Vereecke, L., Beyaert, R. and van Loo, G. (2011) Enterocyte death and intestinal barrier maintenance in homeostasis and disease. Trends Mol. Med. **17**, 584–593

15. Watson, C.J., Oliver, C.H. and Khaled, W.T. (2011) Cytokine signalling in mammary gland development. J. Reprod. Immunol. **88**, 124–129

16. Yu, D. and Turner, J.R. (2008) Stimulus-induced reorganization of tight junction structure: the role of membrane traffic. Biochim. Biophys. Acta **1778**, 709–716

17. Dukes, J.D., Fish, L., Richardson, J.D., Blaikley, E., Burns, S., Caunt, C.J., Chalmers, A.D. and Whitley, P. (2011) Functional ESCRT machinery is required for constitutive recycling of claudin-1 and maintenance of polarity in vertebrate epithelial cells. Mol. Biol. Cell **22**, 3192–3205

18. Dukes, J.D., Whitley, P. and Chalmers, A.D. (2012) The PIKfyve inhibitor YM201636 blocks the continuous recycling of the tight junction proteins claudin-1 and claudin-2 in MDCK cells. PLoS ONE **7**, e28659

19. Morimoto, S., Nishimura, N., Terai, T., Manabe, S., Yamamoto, Y., Shinahara, W., Miyake, H., Tashiro, S., Shimada, M. and Sasaki, T. (2005) Rab13 mediates the continuous endocytic recycling of occludin to the cell surface. J. Biol. Chem. **280**, 2220–2228

20. De Matteis, M.A. and Luini, A. (2008) Exiting the Golgi complex. Nat. Rev. Mol. Cell Biol. **9**, 273–284

21. Welling, P.A. and Weisz, O.A. (2010) Sorting it out in endosomes: an emerging concept in renal epithelial cell transport regulation. Physiology (Bethesda) **25**, 280–292

22. Grant, B.D. and Donaldson, J.G. (2009) Pathways and mechanisms of endocytic recycling. Nat. Rev. Mol. Cell Biol. **10**, 597–608

23. Nishimura, N. and Sasaki, T. (2008) Cell-surface biotinylation to study endocytosis and recycling of occludin. Methods Mol. Biol. **440**, 89–96

24. Takahashi, S., Iwamoto, N., Sasaki, H., Ohashi, M., Oda, Y., Tsukita, S. and Furuse, M. (2009) The E3 ubiquitin ligase LNX1p80 promotes the removal of claudins from tight junctions in MDCK cells. J. Cell Sci. **122**, 985–994

25. McMahon, H.T. and Boucrot, E. (2011) Molecular mechanism and physiological functions of clathrin-mediated endocytosis. Nat. Rev. Mol. Cell Biol. **12**, 517–533

26. Howes, M.T., Mayor, S. and Parton, R.G. (2010) Molecules, mechanisms, and cellular roles of clathrin-independent endocytosis. Curr. Opin. Cell Biol. **22**, 519–527

27. Ivanov, A.I., Nusrat, A. and Parkos, C.A. (2004) Endocytosis of epithelial apical junctional proteins by a clathrin-mediated pathway into a unique storage compartment. Mol. Biol. Cell **15**, 176–188

28. Hopkins, A.M., Walsh, S.V., Verkade, P., Boquet, P. and Nusrat, A. (2003) Constitutive activation of Rho proteins by CNF-1 influences tight junction structure and epithelial barrier function. J. Cell Sci. **116**, 725–742

29. Nighot, P.K. and Blikslager, A.T. (2012) The chloride channel ClC-2 modulates tight junction barrier function via intracellular trafficking of occludin. Am. J. Physiol. Cell Physiol. **302**, C178–C187

30. Bruewer, M., Utech, M., Ivanov, A.I., Hopkins, A.M., Parkos, C.A. and Nusrat, A. (2005) Interferon-γ induces internalization of epithelial tight junction proteins via a macropinocytosis-like process. FASEB J. **19**, 923–933

31. Matsuda, M., Kubo, A., Furuse, M. and Tsukita, S. (2004) A peculiar internalization of claudins, tight junction-specific adhesion molecules, during the intercellular movement of epithelial cells. J. Cell Sci. **117**, 1247–1257

32. Ikari, A., Takiguchi, A., Atomi, K. and Sugatani, J. (2011) Epidermal growth factor increases clathrin-dependent endocytosis and degradation of claudin-2 protein in MDCK II cells. J. Cell Physiol. **226**, 2448–2256

33. Shen, L. and Turner, J.R. (2005) Actin depolymerization disrupts tight junctions via caveolae-mediated endocytosis. Mol. Biol. Cell **16**, 3919–3936

34. Clayburgh, D.R., Barrett, T.A., Tang, Y., Meddings, J.B., Van Eldik, L.J., Watterson, D.M., Clarke, L.L., Mrsny, R.J. and Turner, J.R. (2005) Epithelial myosin light chain kinase-dependent barrier dysfunction mediates T cell activation-induced diarrhea *in vivo*. J. Clin. Invest. **115**, 2702–2715

35. Cummins, P.M. (2012) Occludin: one protein, many forms. Mol. Cell. Biol. **32**, 242–250

36. Findley, M.K. and Koval, M. (2009) Regulation and roles for claudin-family tight junction proteins. IUBMB Life **61**, 431–437

37. Traweger, A., Fang, D., Liu, Y.C., Stelzhammer, W., Krizbai, I.A., Fresser, F., Bauer, H.C. and Bauer, H. (2002) The tight junction-specific protein occludin is a functional target of the E3 ubiquitin-protein ligase itch. J. Biol. Chem. **277**, 10201–10208

38. Banan, A., Zhang, L.J., Shaikh, M., Fields, J.Z., Choudhary, S., Forsyth, C.B., Farhadi, A. and Keshavarzian, A. (2005) theta isoform of protein kinase C alters barrier function in intestinal epithelium through modulation of distinct claudin isotypes: a novel mechanism for regulation of permeability. J. Pharmacol. Exp. Ther. **313**, 962–982

39. Ebnet, K., Aurrand-Lions, M., Kuhn, A., Kiefer, F., Butz, S., Zander, K., Meyer zu Brickwedde, M.K., Suzuki, A., Imhof, B.A. and Vestweber, D. (2003) The junctional adhesion molecule (JAM) family members JAM-2 and JAM-3 associate with the cell polarity protein PAR-3: a possible role for JAMs in endothelial cell polarity. J. Cell Sci. **116**, 3879–3891

40. Raleigh, D.R., Boe, D.M., Yu, D., Weber, C.R., Marchiando, A.M., Bradford, E.M., Wang, Y., Wu, L., Schneeberger, E.E., Shen, L. and Turner, J.R. (2011) Occludin S408 phosphorylation regulates tight junction protein interactions and barrier function. J. Cell Biol. **193**, 565–582

41. Sakakibara, A., Furuse, M., Saitou, M., Ando-Akatsuka, Y. and Tsukita, S. (1997) Possible involvement of phosphorylation of occludin in tight junction formation. J. Cell Biol. **137**, 1393–1401

42. Murakami, T., Felinski, E.A. and Antonetti, D.A. (2009) Occludin phosphorylation and ubiquitination regulate tight junction trafficking and vascular endothelial growth factor-induced permeability. J. Biol. Chem. **284**, 21036–21046

43. Van Itallie, C.M., Gambling, T.M., Carson, J.L. and Anderson, J.M. (2005) Palmitoylation of claudins is required for efficient tight-junction localization. J. Cell Sci. **118**, 1427–1436

44. Abrami, L., Leppla, S.H. and van der Goot, F.G. (2006) Receptor palmitoylation and ubiquitination regulate anthrax toxin endocytosis. J. Cell Biol. **172**, 309–320

45. Kinlough, C.L., McMahan, R.J., Poland, P.A., Bruns, J.B., Harkleroad, K.L., Stremple, R.J., Kashlan, O.B., Weixel, K.M., Weisz, O.A. and Hughey, R.P. (2006) Recycling of MUC1 is dependent on its palmitoylation. J. Biol. Chem. **281**, 12112–12122

46. McCormick, P.J., Dumaresq-Doiron, K., Pluviose, A.S., Pichette, V., Tosato, G. and Lefrancois, S. (2008) Palmitoylation controls recycling in lysosomal sorting and trafficking. Traffic **9**, 1984–1997

47. Shen, L., Weber, C.R. and Turner, J.R. (2008) The tight junction protein complex undergoes rapid and continuous molecular remodeling at steady state. J. Cell Biol. **181**, 683–695

48. Rahner, C., Mitic, L.L. and Anderson, J.M. (2001) Heterogeneity in expression and subcellular localization of claudins 2, 3, 4, and 5 in the rat liver, pancreas, and gut. Gastroenterology **120**, 411–422

49. Van Itallie, C.M., Fanning, A.S. and Anderson, J.M. (2003) Reversal of charge selectivity in cation or anion-selective epithelial lines by expression of different claudins. Am. J. Physiol. Renal Physiol. **285**, F1078–F1084

50. Vogelmann, R. and Nelson, W.J. (2005) Fractionation of the epithelial apical junctional complex: reassessment of protein distributions in different substructures. Mol. Biol. Cell **16**, 701–716

51. Utech, M., Mennigen, R. and Bruewer, M. (2010) Endocytosis and recycling of tight junction proteins in inflammation. J. Biomed. Biotechnol. **2010**, 484987

52. Stamatovic, S.M., Keep, R.F., Wang, M.M., Jankovic, I. and Andjelkovic, A.V. (2009) Caveolae-mediated internalization of occludin and claudin-5 during CCL2-induced tight junction remodeling in brain endothelial cells. J. Biol. Chem. **284**, 19053–19066

53. Hurley, J.H. and Emr, S.D. (2006) The ESCRT complexes: structure and mechanism of a membrane-trafficking network. Annu. Rev. Biophys. Biomol. Struct. **35**, 277–298

54. Raiborg, C. and Stenmark, H. (2009) The ESCRT machinery in endosomal sorting of ubiquitylated membrane proteins. Nature **458**, 445–452

55. Malerod, L., Stuffers, S., Brech, A. and Stenmark, H. (2007) Vps22/EAP30 in ESCRT-II mediates endosomal sorting of growth factor and chemokine receptors destined for lysosomal degradation. Traffic **8**, 1617–1629

56. Baldys, A. and Raymond, J.R. (2009) Critical role of ESCRT machinery in EGFR recycling. Biochemistry **48**, 9321–9323

57. Doyotte, A., Russell, M.R., Hopkins, C.R. and Woodman, P.G. (2005) Depletion of TSG101 forms a mammalian "Class E" compartment: a multicisternal early endosome with multiple sorting defects. J. Cell Sci. **118**, 3003–3017

58. Fujita, H., Yamanaka, M., Imamura, K., Tanaka, Y., Nara, A., Yoshimori, T., Yokota, S. and Himeno, M. (2003) A dominant negative form of the AAA ATPase SKD1/VPS4 impairs membrane trafficking out of endosomal/lysosomal compartments: class E vps phenotype in mammalian cells. J. Cell Sci. **116**, 401–414

59. Yoshimori, T., Yamagata, F., Yamamoto, A., Mizushima, N., Kabeya, Y., Nara, A., Miwako, I., Ohashi, M., Ohsumi, M. and Ohsumi, Y. (2000) The mouse SKD1, a homologue of yeast Vps4p, is required for normal endosomal trafficking and morphology in mammalian cells. Mol. Biol. Cell **11**, 747–763

60. Clague, M.J. and Urbe, S. (2006) Endocytosis: the DUB version. Trends Cell Biol. **16**, 551–559

61. Wright, M.H., Berlin, I. and Nash, P.D. (2011) Regulation of endocytic sorting by ESCRT-DUB-mediated deubiquitination. Cell. Biochem. Biophys. **60**, 39–46

62. de Lartigue, J., Polson, H., Feldman, M., Shokat, K., Tooze, S.A., Urbe, S. and Clague, M.J. (2009) PIKfyve regulation of endosome-linked pathways. Traffic **10**, 883–893

63. Shisheva, A. (2008) PIKfyve: partners, significance, debates and paradoxes. Cell Biol. Int. **32**, 591–604

64. Whitley, P., Reaves, B.J., Hashimoto, M., Riley, A.M., Potter, B.V. and Holman, G.D. (2003) Identification of mammalian Vps24p as an effector of phosphatidylinositol 3,5-bisphosphate-dependent endosome compartmentalization. J. Biol. Chem. **278**, 38786–38795

65. Hutagalung, A.H. and Novick, P.J. (2011) Role of Rab GTPases in membrane traffic and cell physiology. Physiol. Rev. **91**, 119–149

66. Yamamura, R., Nishimura, N., Nakatsuji, H., Arase, S. and Sasaki, T. (2008) The interaction of JRAB/MICAL-L2 with Rab8 and Rab13 coordinates the assembly of tight junctions and adherens junctions. Mol. Biol. Cell **19**, 971–983

67. Nokes, R.L., Fields, I.C., Collins, R.N. and Folsch, H. (2008) Rab13 regulates membrane trafficking between TGN and recycling endosomes in polarized epithelial cells. J. Cell Biol. **182**, 845–853

68. Brennan, K., Offiah, G., McSherry, E.A. and Hopkins, A.M. (2010) Tight junctions: a barrier to the initiation and progression of breast cancer? J. Biomed. Biotechnol. **2010**, 460607

© The Authors Journal compilation © 2012 Biochemical Society
Essays Biochem. (2012) **53**, 55–68: doi: 10.1042/BSE0530055

5

Crucial polarity regulators in axon specification

Giovanna Lalli[1]

Wolfson Centre for Age-Related Diseases, King's College London, Guy's campus, London SE1 1UL, U.K.

Abstract

Cell polarization is critical for the correct functioning of many cell types, creating functional and morphological asymmetry in response to intrinsic and extrinsic cues. Neurons are a classical example of polarized cells, as they usually extend one long axon and short branched dendrites. The formation of such distinct cellular compartments (also known as neuronal polarization) ensures the proper development and physiology of the nervous system and is controlled by a complex set of signalling pathways able to integrate multiple polarity cues. Because polarization is at the basis of neuronal development, investigating the mechanisms responsible for this process is fundamental not only to understand how the nervous system develops, but also to devise therapeutic strategies for neuroregeneration. The last two decades have seen remarkable progress in understanding the molecular mechanisms responsible for mammalian neuronal polarization, primarily using cultures of rodent hippocampal neurons. More recent efforts have started to explore the role of such mechanisms *in vivo*. It has become clear that neuronal polarization relies on signalling networks and feedback mechanisms co-ordinating the actin and microtubule cytoskeleton and membrane traffic. The present chapter will highlight the role of key molecules involved in neuronal polarization, such as regulators of the actin/microtubule cytoskeleton and membrane traffic, polarity complexes and small GTPases.

[1]*giovanna.lalli@kcl.ac.uk*

Introduction

The polarization of neurons into axonal and dendritic compartments is a fundamental event for their development. Disruption of this process impairs the directional signalling between neurons, thus severely compromising their function. From the clinical point of view, studying the molecular mechanisms that underlie axon specification and growth is crucial if we hope to restore neuronal function in injury or neurodegenerative diseases. Indeed, recent studies *in vitro* have demonstrated the ability of old mature neurons to reactivate an intrinsic polarization programme favouring axon regrowth after lesion [1], an event that could be the key to regeneration in the nervous system after trauma, injury or in degenerative diseases.

Neuronal polarization relies on the fine regulation of cytoskeletal dynamics and membrane traffic. Over the last two decades many studies have investigated this process using cultured embryonic hippocampal neurons [2]. These cells develop through stereotyped stages, culminating in the clear compartmentalization of axon and dendrites (Figure 1). Immediately after plating, neurons are round and extend dynamic lamellipodia and filopodia (stage 1). This is followed by the extension of multiple short neurites (stage 2). Approximately half a day after plating (stage 3), one of these neurites starts to grow [3] and becomes the nascent axon. This will continue to elongate in the following 4–7 days while the rest of the neurites mature into dendrites (stage 4) and subsequently display spines (stage 5). In the present chapter I will focus on some molecular players crucial for axon specification, including regulators of the cytoskeleton, crucial signalling pathways and small GTPases. For more in-depth analysis of different aspects involved in neuronal polarization I refer the reader to excellent reviews [4–6].

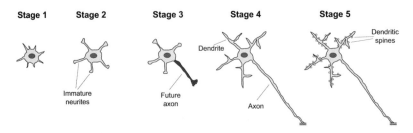

Figure 1. Hippocampal neuron polarization *in vitro*
In stage 1, round neurons display dynamic lamellipodial and filopodial activity. In stage 2, they extend multiple immature neurites. In stage 3, one of these neurites starts to grow rapidly. Microtubule stabilization in the shaft (dark blue) and enhanced microtubule/actin dynamics at the growth cone of the future axon (red) play a key role in this crucial polarization step. In stage 4, the minor neurites mature into dendrites, whereas the axon extends and branches. Finally, in stage 5, dendrites display spines (yellow) to establish functional synapses.

The cytoskeleton

The cytoskeleton is a key player in neuronal polarization. A close interaction between actin filaments and microtubules (Figure 2, red and turquoise respectively) is observed in the growth cone, an important structure at the tip of the presumptive axon. Microtubules stabilize the nascent axon shaft and grow until the C-domain (central domain) of the growth cone (white background in Figure 2), helping the transport of vesicles and organelles towards the leading edge. In the growth cone peripheral area (also known as the 'P-domain', yellow background in Figure 2), filopodia (bundles of actin filaments) dynamically extend and retract, sensing the extracellular environment through receptors and providing directionality to axon growth. These filopodia are connected by thin lamellipodia, structures formed by an intricate actin filament meshwork [7]. Actin filaments forming filopodia and lamellipodia in the P-domain point their depolymerizing end towards the narrow region at the border between the C- and P-domains, the so-called T-zone (transition zone, purple background in Figure 2), whereas their fast growing ends are oriented towards the distal membrane. The 'push' of actin polymerization towards the periphery, together with the contractile action of the actin-driven motor myosin II anchored at the T-zone drives continuous movement of F-actin (filamentous actin) from the leading edge towards the centre of the growth cone. This process is called F-actin 'retrograde

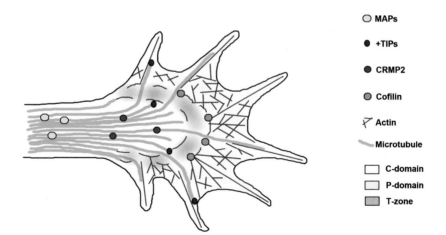

Figure 2. Schematic organization of the growth cone at the axon tip
Microtubules (turquoise) grow towards the C-domain of the growth cone (white background). During polarization, MAPs (yellow) stabilize the shaft of the future axon. CRMP2 (pink) can favour microtubule polymerization and endocytosis (see the text for details). +TIPs (blue) and APC bind to the plus-ends of microtubules, stabilizing them. They may also provide a link with the actin cytoskeleton (red). Actin arcs and depolymerization of actin filaments (red) favoured by cofilin (orange) are observed in the T-zone (purple background). Dynamic filopodia and lamellipodia are found in the P-domain (yellow background) together with some microtubules able to get through the T-zone and extend along filopodia.

flow'. Contraction of actin filaments by myosin II in the T-zone also leads to the formation of 'actin arcs', which are oriented perpendicular to the peripheral filopodia. Although actin arcs block microtubule growth into the P-domain [7], it is possible to observe some microtubules extending until the very end of filopodia [8]. Axon extension is favoured by actin depolymerization at the neck of the growth cone, which allows microtubule invasion of the C-domain and bundling, causing the consolidation of the proximal part of the growth cone and its transformation into a new segment of axon shaft. Such close interplay between the actin and microtubule cytoskeleton is critical for axon formation and needs to be precisely controlled.

Actin dynamics

Local actin depolymerization in one of the initial neurites is sufficient to promote or even regenerate axon growth [9]. Therefore, to allow microtubule extension, the actin cytoskeleton in the growth cone of the future axon has to be much more dynamic than in the minor neurites. Consistent with this idea, several regulators of actin dynamics are involved in neuronal polarization, at least *in vitro*: these include the WAVE [WASP (Wiskott–Aldrich syndrome protein) verprolin homologous] complex [10] and cofilin [11]. The WAVE complex regulates actin polymerization in lamellipodia [12], whereas cofilin binds to the minus ends of the actin filaments, favouring their severing and depolymerization. Expression of non-functional WAVE or inhibition of WAVE transport into the axon blocks axon growth in hippocampal and cerebellar granule neurons [10,13]. In addition, a conditional knockout mouse model for Cdc42 (cell division cycle 42), a small GTPase involved in the control of filopodia formation and polarity (see also below), displays strong neuronal polarity defects caused at least, in part, by increased levels of phosphorylated (inactive) cofilin. Depolymerizing actin filaments rescued axon formation in Cdc42-depleted neurons, consistent with a requirement for a dynamic actin cytoskeleton in the establishment of polarity [11].

Microtubule dynamics

The initial growth of an axon relies on the consolidation and bundling of microtubules, so that the C-domain of the growth cone becomes part of the axon shaft. Microtubules consist of tubulin heterodimers, which polymerize with the plus-end oriented towards the axon tip. This location is characterized by 'dynamic instability', that is cycles of rapid microtubule assembly and disassembly ('shrinkage'). The switch from growth to shrinkage is instead known as 'catastrophe' [14]. Importantly, microtubules have an instructive role in axon specification. In contrast with actin, microtubules in the axon are more stable compared with other neurites. Indeed, modest pharmacological microtubule stabilization that prevents catastrophe without completely blocking microtubule growth produces supernumerary axons *in vitro* [15]. Moreover, local microtubule stabilization of one minor neurite causes it to become an axon, a remarkable phenomenon also observed with dendrites in mature neurons [1], suggesting that the potential to switch fate and extend as an axon is also maintained at later stages.

Post-translational tubulin modifications, such as detyrosination and acetylation, characterize stable microtubules and are found in the proximal section of the axon, in contrast with the C-domain of the axonal growth cone, where more dynamic microtubules prevail to quickly rearrange in response to extracellular guidance cues. The plus-end-directed motor KIF5 (kinesin-5) binds acetylated (stable) microtubules and preferentially accumulates in one neurite before morphological polarization, favouring transport of organelles and cargo into the nascent axon [16]. Its activity is required for axon specification, since dominant-negative KIF5 or KIF5 depletion impair neuronal polarization [17]. Although it is clear that regulation of microtubule dynamics is crucial for neuronal polarization, it will be important to investigate further how post-translational modifications of tubulin and motor proteins can be controlled to ensure microtubule consolidation and polarized transport in the perspective axon [18].

MAPs (microtubule-associated proteins)

Regulators of microtubule stability play an important role in axon specification, these include traditional MAPs belonging to the MAP2/tau family [19]. A crucial MAP in neuronal polarity is CRMP2 (collapsin-response-mediator protein 2). Overexpression of CRMP2 results in multiple axons, whereas dominant-negative CRMP2 impairs axon specification [20]. Importantly, overexpression of CRMP2 also causes a stage 4 dendrite to become an axon, suggesting that CRMP2 is sufficient to switch the fate not only of immature neurites, but also of mature dendrites [20]. CRMP2 may perform several important functions related to polarization. First, it carries tubulin heterodimers, favouring microtubule assembly. Secondly, it promotes transport of the actin-remodelling Sra-1 (specifically Rac1-associated protein 1)–WAVE complex along microtubules by linking it to the motor protein kinesin-1. Proper localization of the Sra-1–WAVE complex (which regulates actin stability during lamellipodia formation) is important for neuronal polarization since knockdown of Sra-1 or WAVE prevents CRMP2-dependent axon formation. Finally, CRMP-2 specifically accumulates in the C-domain where it binds Numb (a protein involved in clathrin-mediated endocytosis) and regulates endocytosis of L1, a neuronal cell-adhesion molecule important for axon growth [21].

+TIPs (plus-end tracking proteins)

+TIPs regulate microtubule dynamics by binding to the plus-end of microtubules where polymerization occurs. The +TIP CLIPs (cytoplasmic linker proteins) 170 and 115 favour the switch from microtubule catastrophe to polymerization, an important event in axon specification. Transfection of dominant-negative CLIPs impairs neuronal polarization, whereas overexpression of their microtubule-binding domains produces supernumerary axons, suggesting that

CLIPs are sufficient for polarization [22]. Why multiple homologues of CLIPs exist, how their function is regulated and whether their role is conserved *in vivo* remains to be investigated.

Similar to CLIPs, the APC (adenomatous polyposis coli) protein also accumulates at microtubule plus-ends and concentrates at the tip of the presumptive axon in stage 3 neurons, increasing microtubule stability. Overexpressing truncated forms of APC or depleting APC impairs neuronal polarization in mammalian neurons *in vitro* [23,24]; however, work in *Drosophila* suggests that APC may be dispensable for axon specification [25]. More studies will be needed to clarify whether APC is necessary for neuronal polarization *in vivo*. Interestingly, CLIPs and APC contain a domain able to directly interact with the actin cytoskeleton [26,27], potentially mediating cross-talk between the growing microtubule ends and the actin cortex. Indeed, recent observations raise the possibility that the mutual influence of the actin network and the microtubule cytoskeleton are part of a positive-feedback loop involved in establishing an axon by controlling growth cone dynamics [5]. The molecular nature of the microtubule–actin relationship in the growing axon still has to be completely elucidated. Such a relationship, however, is very likely to also maintain a central role in neuronal polarization *in vivo*.

Intracellular signalling

PI3K (phosphoinositide 3-kinase)/Akt/GSK3 (glycogen synthase kinase 3)

The lipid kinase PI3K, an effector of the small GTPase Ras, produces localized enrichment of PtdIns(3,4,5)P_3 at the membrane. Several studies indicate that PI3K activity is both necessary and sufficient for axon formation, since PI3K inhibition prevents axon specification, whereas overexpression of a constitutively active catalytic subunit of PI3K causes multiple axons [28–30]. PI3K activity is counteracted by PTEN (phosphatase and tensin homologue deleted on chromosome 10), a protein and lipid phosphatase that dephosphorylates PtdIns(3,4,5)P_3 into PtdIns(4,5)P_2, thus counteracting PtdIns(3,4,5)P_3 signalling. Overexpression of PTEN prevents axon specification [28], whereas PTEN depletion leads to multiple axons [31], thus demonstrating the requirement of tightly controlled PtdIns(3,4,5)P_3 levels for axon specification.

PI3K triggers a cascade of effects (Figure 3, right-hand side), such as activation of Rap1b [32], a small GTPase necessary and sufficient for neuronal polarization (see below) [33] and of the protein kinase Akt, recruited by its PH (pleckstrin homology) domain to PtdIns(3,4,5)P_3-enriched sites. Akt can subsequently phosphorylate and inhibit GSK3, a key regulator of neuronal polarization [31]. The most important effect of GSK3 inhibition is the activation of microtubule-binding proteins normally suppressed by GSK3, such as CRMP2, APC, MAP1b and tau [21], resulting in microtubule stabilization. How the action of these multiple GSK3 effectors is then co-ordinated during

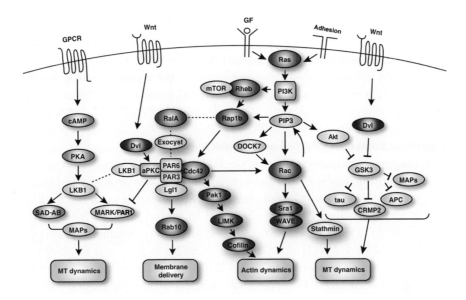

Figure 3. Key intracellular signalling pathways in neuronal polarization
Small GTPases of the Rho, Ras and Rab families (pink) regulate neuronal polarization by influencing microtubule/actin dynamics and membrane traffic. Downstream of a variety of extracellular factors Ras activates PI3K causing a localized increase of PtdIns(3,4,5)P_3 at the membrane (right-hand side). This leads to a cascade of events, including activation of the Akt/GSK3 pathway and Rac regulating the cytoskeleton, Rheb influencing translation, and Rap1b and Cdc42 regulating actin dynamics and localization of the PAR-3–PAR-6–aPKC complex. The PAR complex affects the actin cytoskeleton via Rac, microtubule dynamics via MARK and membrane delivery via Lgl1. Correct localization of the PAR complex is ensured by local activation of RalA and the exocyst complex. The PAR family member LKB1 acts downstream of the cAMP/PKA pathway (left-hand side), controlling microtubule dynamics via MARKs and SAD kinase activation. From non-neuronal studies LKB1 has the potential to interact with the PAR complex; however, it is still unclear whether this interaction has a role in neuronal polarity. The Wnt pathway may regulate polarity via Dvl by activating aPKC and/or inhibiting GSK3. See the text for details. GF, growth factor; GPCR, G-protein-coupled receptor; LIMK, LIM kinase; MT, microtubule; mTOR, mammalian target of rapamycin; PIP3, PtdIns(3,4,5)P_3.

axon specification remains to be understood. Surprisingly, double knock-in mice lacking the Akt phosphorylation sites in both GSK3 isoforms exhibit normal axon polarity *in vivo* [34], suggesting the existence of different modes of GSK3 inhibition not requiring Akt-dependent phosphorylation. These may include the Wnt signalling pathway, which can indirectly inhibit GSK3 via the Frizzled receptor and Dvl (Dishevelled). Interestingly, Wnt5a activates Dvl, which in turn binds and activates aPKC (atypical protein kinase C) [35]. The final result is aPKC-dependent phosphorylation and inhibition of the microtubule-destabilizing protein MARK (MAP-regulating kinase) 2/PAR (PARtitioning defective)-1 [36] (see below), which favours growth of the future axon.

PAR family members

The six PAR genes were originally identified in a genetic screen to identify regulators of asymmetric cell division in *Caenorhabditis elegans* [37] and are known to play a pivotal role in many polarization events, such as asymmetric mitotic spindle positioning, polarized localization of fate determinants and epithelial cell polarization throughout metazoans [38]. Some PAR family members are also involved in neuronal polarity: they include the serine/threonine kinases PAR-1 and PAR-4, and the scaffold proteins PAR-3 and PAR-6 (Figure 3, left-hand side).

LKB1(liver kinase B1)/PAR-4 and MARKs

LKB1 (the mammalian orthologue of the *PAR4* gene) is a key regulator of neuronal polarization, both *in vitro* and *in vivo* [39,40]. Once activated by binding to its necessary co-activator Strad and by phosphorylation on Ser^{431} by PKA (protein kinase A) or p90[RSK] (p90 ribosomal S6 kinase) kinases [39,40], LKB1 phosphorylates a variety of substrates including the mammalian orthologues of PAR-1 (MARK1–4) [41]. Among these, MARK2 may act as a negative regulator of neuronal polarization since its depletion causes multiple axons [36]. LKB1-activated MARK2 phosphorylates a range of MAPs, causing them to detach from microtubules and leading to microtubule destabilization. LKB1 may favour MARK2 activation to promote local microtubule instability in the growth cone of the nascent axon, whereas other factors may inactivate MARK2 to stabilize microtubules in the axon shaft [41]. LKB1 also activates SAD (synapses of the amphid defective)-A/B kinases, which phosphorylate and modulate the microtubule-binding affinity of several MAPs, including MAP2, MAP4 and tau [4,41]. These effects ultimately modify microtubule organization to favour axon formation. Depletion of SAD kinases partially blocks the multiple axon phenotype caused by LKB1 overexpression, showing that LKB1 can influence axon specification, at least in part, by phosphorylating SAD kinases [39]. Besides affecting MAPs, it is tempting to speculate that SAD kinases may also function in promoting directed vesicular traffic along the axon, given their ability to promote presynaptic vesicular clustering in *C. elegans* [42].

The PAR-3–PAR-6–aPKC complex

PAR-3 and PAR-6 localize at the tip of the nascent axon in stage 3 neurons and their depletion inhibits polarization, whereas overexpression of PAR-3 causes multiple axon formation [28]. PAR-3 and PAR-6 associate with aPKC and inhibit its activity. However, localized activation of the small GTPase Cdc42 (see below), which binds to PAR-6, relieves this inhibition, achieving local and temporal control of aPKC activity [4]. aPKC subsequently phosphorylates some crucial targets, such as Lgl1 (lethal giant larvae 1), a PAR-3/6 binding partner involved in various polarization events, such as asymmetric cell division and polarized membrane traffic in neuroblasts and epithelia. Lgl1 in turn activates Rab10, a Rab GTPase promoting polarized membrane insertion, a process required for axonal specification *in vitro* and *in vivo* [43].

aPKC in complex with PAR-3–PAR-6 can also phosphorylate and inactivate MARKs, such as MARK2, leading to MAP dephosphorylation and microtubule stabilization in the nascent axon [36]. Finally, the active Cdc42–PAR–aPKC complex also acts as an important scaffold platform to locally recruit activators of small GTPases such as the Rac GEFs (guanine-nucleotide-exchange factors) Tiam1 (T-cell lymphoma invasion and metastasis 1) and STEF (Sif and Tiam1-like exchange factor), ultimately influencing microtubule and actin dynamics at the axonal tip [44] (also see below). Interestingly, in *Drosophila* the PAR complex does not appear to be needed for axonogenesis [45]. This could be due to a species-specific requirement, even though formal confirmation of a role for PAR-3 and PAR-6 in neuronal polarization *in vivo* is still needed in mammalian systems.

Small GTPases

Several GTPases control neuronal polarization through their ability to influence cytoskeletal dynamics, protein translation and membrane traffic [46]. They are molecular switches, cycling between an active GTP-bound state, and an inactive GDP-bound state. GEFs activate GTPases by mediating the exchange of GDP for GTP, whereas GAPs (GTPase-activating proteins) inactivate them by stimulating their intrinsic GTPase activity. Interaction with specific effectors and a tight spatial/temporal control of GTPase activation can be achieved by the localized action of GEFs and GAPs, which is also observed in neuronal polarization.

Growth factor signalling and extracellular matrix signals can activate several members of the Ras GTPase family, including H-Ras, R-Ras, K-Ras and N-Ras (Figure 3). Polarized localization of R-Ras in one neurite is already visible in stage 2 [5,47], and is maintained by a positive-feedback loop involving the Ras effector PI3K [48]. This produces $PtdIns(3,4,5)P_3$ in the nascent axon and, as a consequence, leads to activation of kinases such as integrin-linked kinase and Akt, both of which are able to inactivate GSK3, leading to microtubule stabilization (see above). In addition, $PtdIns(3,4,5)P_3$ helps to localize the Rac GEF DOCK (dedicator of cytokinesis protein) 7 to the membrane of the nascent axon via its DHR-1 (DOCK homology region 1) domain. Activation of the small Rho GTPase Rac regulates local actin dynamics and lamellipodia formation, but can also lead to phosphorylation and inhibition of stathmin, a microtubule-destabilizing molecule, thus favouring axon growth [49]. In addition, Rac participates in a positive-feedback loop by activating PI3K [21], which would reinforce a localized signalling pathway promoting axonogenesis at the tip of the future axon. Here, active Cdc42, together with the PAR–aPKC complex, promotes local activation of Rac thanks to the ability of PAR-3 to directly interact with and recruit the Rac GEFs Tiam1 or STEF. Indeed, overexpression of Tiam1 leads to multiple axons, whereas its depletion impairs neuronal polarization [44]. Overall, these observations support an important role for Rac in axonogenesis; however, Rac1 RNAi (RNA interference) in both *Drosophila* and mammalian neurons does not seem to affect neuronal polarity [4]. It is likely that other Rac isoforms, such as Rac3, may be able to compensate for Rac1 depletion.

Another Ras family member, the small GTPase Rheb, and its target mTOR (mammalian target of rapamycin) also operate downstream of PI3K [50] by increasing translation of the Ras-related GTPase Rap1b in the nascent axon. Rap1b plays a pivotal role in neuronal polarity *in vitro*, since its depletion impairs axonogenesis, whereas its overexpression leads to multiple axons [33]. The small GTPase Cdc42, a master polarity regulator, also has a central role in axon specification. Both dominant-negative and constitutively active Cdc42 versions block axon specification, whereas transfection of a 'fast-cycling' mutant, which autonomously cycles between a GDP- and a GTP-bound state, produces a multiple axon phenotype and rescues the loss of axons due to Rap1b depletion, placing Cdc42 downstream of Rap1b [33]. This highlights the importance of a tight regulation of GTPase cycling in the nascent axon. The necessary role for Cdc42 in neuronal polarity has been shown *in vivo* with a conditional knockout mouse model displaying severe axonogenesis defects [11]. These may be due to alteration in actin dynamics, as suggested by abnormally high levels of phosphorylated cofilin, a substrate for LIM kinase, which can be activated by the Cdc42 effector Pak-1 (p21-activated kinase-1). Pak-1 is enriched in the presumptive axon in stage 3 neurons and is necessary and sufficient for neuronal polarization [51]. In addition to regulating actin dynamics, Cdc42 favours polarization by binding to PAR-6 and activating the PAR–aPKC polarity complex at the axon tip, triggering a series of downstream events culminating in microtubule stabilization (see the previous section on PAR).

Finally, the Ras-like GTPase RalA regulates neuronal polarity through the exocyst, a protein complex involved in several polarization events, such as bud growth in yeast, basolateral membrane delivery in epithelial cells and directed cell migration [52]. RalA is likely to act downstream of Rap1b, since Rap can activate RalGEFs in non-neuronal cells. Similar to the PAR complex, the exocyst accumulates at the tip of the future axon in stage 3 neurons. Importantly, biochemical evidence shows a progressive interaction between the exocyst and the PAR complex as polarization occurs, and such interaction depends on RalA activation [53]. Although the nature of this interaction still has to be clarified, it is interesting to note that depletion of either RalA or multiple exocyst subunits impairs the polarized localization of the PAR complex, and, as a consequence, inhibits neuronal polarization.

Conclusion

The last two decades have highlighted the role of many key players and signalling pathways in neuronal polarity. We are now left with a number of unanswered questions concerning the validity of these findings in a more physiological context. Do such signalling cascades also control neuronal polarity *in vivo*? Genetic manipulation, together with the latest advances in time-lapse imaging technology will help to answer this question. Also, how can extracellular cues and intrinsic cell polarity pathways integrate to achieve spatial and temporal control of polarization in different neuronal cell types? And finally, how is the interplay between cytoskeletal dynamics and membrane traffic co-ordinated at a molecular level? Tackling these challenging questions will clarify not only how a neuron develops its polarized morphology, but also how this process may be exploited in regenerative strategies.

Summary

- *Neuronal polarity relies on the co-ordinated interplay between the actin and microtubule cytoskeleton, polarized membrane traffic and regulated protein translation.*
- *Polarized activation of PI3K and local enrichment of its product PtdIns(3,4,5)P_3 are required for axon specification.*
- *Inhibition of GSK3 is a key event in neuronal polarity, leading to microtubule stabilization in the growing axon.*
- *The Cdc42–PAR-3–PAR-6–aPKC complex acts as a central signalling scaffold contributing to the control of actin/microtubule dynamics and membrane traffic in the perspective axon.*
- *LKB1 (PAR-4) is a crucial regulator of neuronal polarization by phosphorylating SAD-A/B kinases and MARK2 (PAR-1), ultimately affecting microtubule dynamics in the nascent axon.*
- *The small GTPase Ras may act upstream of signalling cascades involving other GTPases, such as Rap1b, Cdc42, RalA, Rac and Rheb, all required for axon specification.*

I apologize to all of the authors whose work could not be cited due to space limitation. I thank Giovanni Lesa for valuable comments and discussions. This work was supported by King's College London and by the Wellcome Trust.

References

1. Gomis-Ruth, S., Wierenga, C.J. and Bradke, F. (2008) Plasticity of polarization: changing dendrites into axons in neurons integrated in neuronal circuits. Curr. Biol. **18**, 992–1000
2. Dotti, C.G., Sullivan, C.A. and Banker, G.A. (1988) The establishment of polarity by hippocampal neurons in culture. J. Neurosci. **8**, 1454–1468
3. Bradke, F. and Dotti, C.G. (1997) Neuronal polarity: vectorial cytoplasmic flow precedes axon formation. Neuron **19**, 1175–1186
4. Barnes, A.P. and Polleux, F. (2009) Establishment of axon-dendrite polarity in developing neurons. Annu. Rev. Neurosci. **32**, 347–381
5. Neukirchen, D. and Bradke, F. (2011) Neuronal polarization and the cytoskeleton. Semin. Cell Dev. Biol. **22**, 825–833
6. Polleux, F. and Snider, W. (2010) Initiating and growing an axon. Cold Spring Harb. Persp. Biol. **2**, a001925
7. Lowery, L.A. and Van Vactor, D. (2009) The trip of the tip: understanding the growth cone machinery. Nat. Rev. Mol. Cell Biol. **10**, 332–343

8.   Dent, E.W., Gupton, S.L. and Gertler, F.B. (2011) The growth cone cytoskeleton in axon outgrowth and guidance. Cold Spring Harb. Persp. Biol. **3**, a001800

9.   Bradke, F. and Dotti, C.G. (1999) The role of local actin instability in axon formation. Science **283**, 1931–1934

10. Tahirovic, S., Hellal, F., Neukirchen, D., Hindges, R., Garvalov, B.K., Flynn, K.C., Stradal, T.E., Chrostek-Grashoff, A., Brakebusch, C. and Bradke, F. (2010) Rac1 regulates neuronal polarization through the WAVE complex. J. Neurosci. **30**, 6930–6943

11. Garvalov, B.K., Flynn, K.C., Neukirchen, D., Meyn, L., Teusch, N., Wu, X., Brakebusch, C., Bamburg, J.R. and Bradke, F. (2007) Cdc42 regulates cofilin during the establishment of neuronal polarity. J. Neurosci. **27**, 13117–13129

12. Takenawa, T. and Suetsugu, S. (2007) The WASP-WAVE protein network: connecting the membrane to the cytoskeleton. Nat. Rev. Mol. Cell Biol. **8**, 37–48

13. Arimura, N., Menager, C., Kawano, Y., Yoshimura, T., Kawabata, S., Hattori, A., Fukata, Y., Amano, M., Goshima, Y., Inagaki, M. et al. (2005) Phosphorylation by Rho kinase regulates CRMP-2 activity in growth cones. Mol. Cell Biol. **25**, 9973–9984

14. Howard, J. and Hyman, A.A. (2003) Dynamics and mechanics of the microtubule plus end. Nature **422**, 753–758

15. Witte, H., Neukirchen, D. and Bradke, F. (2008) Microtubule stabilization specifies initial neuronal polarization. J. Cell Biol. **180**, 619–632

16. Jacobson, C., Schnapp, B. and Banker, G.A. (2006) A change in the selective translocation of the kinesin-1 motor domain marks the initial specification of the axon. Neuron **49**, 797–804

17. Kimura, T., Watanabe, H., Iwamatsu, A. and Kaibuchi, K. (2005) Tubulin and CRMP-2 complex is transported via kinesin-1. J. Neurochem. **93**, 1371–1382

18. Hammond, J.W., Huang, C.F., Kaech, S., Jacobson, C., Banker, G. and Verhey, K.J. (2010) Posttranslational modifications of tubulin and the polarized transport of kinesin-1 in neurons. Mol. Biol. Cell **21**, 572–583

19. Conde, C. and Caceres, A. (2009) Microtubule assembly, organization and dynamics in axons and dendrites. Nat. Rev. Neurosci. **10**, 319–332

20. Inagaki, N., Chihara, K., Arimura, N., Menager, C., Kawano, Y., Matsuo, N., Nishimura, T., Amano, M. and Kaibuchi, K. (2001) CRMP-2 induces axons in cultured hippocampal neurons. Nat. Neurosci. **4**, 781–782

21. Arimura, N. and Kaibuchi, K. (2007) Neuronal polarity: from extracellular signals to intracellular mechanisms. Nat. Rev. Neurosci. **8**, 194–205

22. Neukirchen, D. and Bradke, F. (2011) Cytoplasmic linker proteins regulate neuronal polarization through microtubule and growth cone dynamics. J. Neurosci. **31**, 1528–1538

23. Shi, S.H., Cheng, T., Jan, L.Y. and Jan, Y.N. (2004) APC and GSK-3β are involved in mPar3 targeting to the nascent axon and establishment of neuronal polarity. Curr. Biol. **14**, 2025–2032

24. Zhou, F.Q., Zhou, J., Dedhar, S., Wu, Y.H. and Snider, W.D. (2004) NGF-induced axon growth is mediated by localized inactivation of GSK-3β and functions of the microtubule plus end binding protein APC. Neuron **42**, 897–912

25. Rusan, N.M., Akong, K. and Peifer, M. (2008) Putting the model to the test: are APC proteins essential for neuronal polarity, axon outgrowth, and axon targeting? J. Cell Biol. **183**, 203–212

26. Moseley, J.B., Bartolini, F., Okada, K., Wen, Y., Gundersen, G.G. and Goode, B.L. (2007) Regulated binding of adenomatous polyposis coli protein to actin. J. Biol. Chem. **282**, 12661–12668

27. Tsvetkov, A.S., Samsonov, A., Akhmanova, A., Galjart, N. and Popov, S.V. (2007) Microtubule-binding proteins CLASP1 and CLASP2 interact with actin filaments. Cell Motil. Cytoskeleton **64**, 519–530

28. Shi, S.H., Jan, L.Y. and Jan, Y.N. (2003) Hippocampal neuronal polarity specified by spatially localized mPar3/mPar6 and PI 3-kinase activity. Cell **112**, 63–75

29. Menager, C., Arimura, N., Fukata, Y. and Kaibuchi, K. (2004) PIP3 is involved in neuronal polarization and axon formation. J. Neurochem. **89**, 109–118

30. Yoshimura, T., Arimura, N., Kawano, Y., Kawabata, S., Wang, S. and Kaibuchi, K. (2006) Ras regulates neuronal polarity via the PI3-kinase/Akt/GSK-3beta/CRMP-2 pathway. Biochem. Biophys. Res. Commun. **340**, 62–68

31. Jiang, H., Guo, W., Liang, X. and Rao, Y. (2005) Both the establishment and the maintenance of neuronal polarity require active mechanisms: critical roles of GSK-3β and its upstream regulators. Cell **120**, 123–135

32. Bos, J.L., de Rooij, J. and Reedquist, K.A. (2001) Rap1 signalling: adhering to new models. Nat. Rev. Mol. Cell Biol. **2**, 369–377

33. Schwamborn, J.C. and Puschel, A.W. (2004) The sequential activity of the GTPases Rap1B and Cdc42 determines neuronal polarity. Nat. Neurosci. **7**, 923–929

34. Gartner, A., Huang, X. and Hall, A. (2006) Neuronal polarity is regulated by glycogen synthase kinase-3 (GSK-3β) independently of Akt/PKB serine phosphorylation. J. Cell Sci. **119**, 3927–3934

35. Zhang, X., Zhu, J., Yang, G.Y., Wang, Q.J., Qian, L., Chen, Y.M., Chen, F., Tao, Y., Hu, H.S., Wang, T. and Luo, Z.G. (2007) Dishevelled promotes axon differentiation by regulating atypical protein kinase C. Nat. Cell Biol. **9**, 743–754

36. Chen, Y.M., Wang, Q.J., Hu, H.S., Yu, P.C., Zhu, J., Drewes, G., Piwnica-Worms, H. and Luo, Z.G. (2006) Microtubule affinity-regulating kinase 2 functions downstream of the PAR-3/PAR-6/atypical PKC complex in regulating hippocampal neuronal polarity. Proc. Natl. Acad. Sci. U.S.A. **103**, 8534–8539

37. Kemphues, K.J., Priess, J.R., Morton, D.G. and Cheng, N.S. (1988) Identification of genes required for cytoplasmic localization in early *C. elegans* embryos. Cell **52**, 311–320

38. Insolera, R., Chen, S. and Shi, S.H. (2011) Par proteins and neuronal polarity. Dev. Neurobiol. **71**, 483–494

39. Barnes, A.P., Lilley, B.N., Pan, Y.A., Plummer, L.J., Powell, A.W., Raines, A.N., Sanes, J.R. and Polleux, F. (2007) LKB1 and SAD kinases define a pathway required for the polarization of cortical neurons. Cell **129**, 549–563

40. Shelly, M., Cancedda, L., Heilshorn, S., Sumbre, G. and Poo, M.M. (2007) LKB1/STRAD promotes axon initiation during neuronal polarization. Cell **129**, 565–577

41. Shelly, M. and Poo, M.M. (2011) Role of LKB1-SAD/MARK pathway in neuronal polarization. Dev. Neurobiol. **71**, 508–527

42. Crump, J.G., Zhen, M., Jin, Y. and Bargmann, C.I. (2001) The SAD-1 kinase regulates presynaptic vesicle clustering and axon termination. Neuron **29**, 115–129

43. Wang, T., Liu, Y., Xu, X.H., Deng, C.Y., Wu, K.Y., Zhu, J., Fu, X.Q., He, M. and Luo, Z.G. (2011) Lgl1 activation of rab10 promotes axonal membrane trafficking underlying neuronal polarization. Dev. Cell **21**, 431–444

44. Nishimura, T., Yamaguchi, T., Kato, K., Yoshizawa, M., Nabeshima, Y., Ohno, S., Hoshino, M. and Kaibuchi, K. (2005) PAR-6-PAR-3 mediates Cdc42-induced Rac activation through the Rac GEFs STEF/Tiam1. Nat. Cell Biol. **7**, 270–277

45. Rolls, M.M. and Doe, C.Q. (2004) Baz, Par-6 and aPKC are not required for axon or dendrite specification in *Drosophila*. Nat. Neurosci. **7**, 1293–1295

46. Hall, A. and Lalli, G. (2010) Rho and Ras GTPases in axon growth, guidance, and branching. Cold Spring Harb. Perspect. Biol. **2**, a001818

47. Oinuma, I., Katoh, H. and Negishi, M. (2007) R-Ras controls axon specification upstream of glycogen synthase kinase-3β through integrin-linked kinase. J. Biol. Chem. **282**, 303–318

48. Fivaz, M., Bandara, S., Inoue, T. and Meyer, T. (2008) Robust neuronal symmetry breaking by Ras-triggered local positive feedback. Curr. Biol. **18**, 44–50

49. Watabe-Uchida, M., John, K.A., Janas, J.A., Newey, S.E. and Van Aelst, L. (2006) The Rac activator DOCK7 regulates neuronal polarity through local phosphorylation of stathmin/Op18. Neuron **51**, 727–739

50. Li, Y.H., Werner, H. and Puschel, A.W. (2008) Rheb and mTOR regulate neuronal polarity through Rap1B. J. Biol. Chem. **283**, 33784–33792

51. Jacobs, T., Causeret, F., Nishimura, Y.V., Terao, M., Norman, A., Hoshino, M. and Nikolic, M. (2007) Localized activation of p21-activated kinase controls neuronal polarity and morphology. J. Neurosci. **27**, 8604–8615

52. He, B. and Guo, W. (2009) The exocyst complex in polarized exocytosis. Curr. Opin. Cell Biol. **21**, 537–542

53. Lalli, G. (2009) RalA and the exocyst complex influence neuronal polarity through PAR-3 and aPKC. J. Cell Sci. **122**, 1499–1506

© The Authors Journal compilation © 2012 Biochemical Society
Essays Biochem. (2012) **53**, 69–82: doi: 10.1042/BSE0530069

6

Cell wars: regulation of cell survival and proliferation by cell competition

Silvia Vivarelli[1], Laura Wagstaff[1] and Eugenia Piddini[2]

The Wellcome Trust/Cancer Research UK Gurdon Institute, University of Cambridge, Tennis Court Road, Cambridge CB2 1QN, U.K.

Abstract

During cell competition fitter cells take over the tissue at the expense of viable, but less fit, cells, which are eliminated by induction of apoptosis or senescence. This probably acts as a quality-control mechanism to eliminate suboptimal cells and safeguard organ function. Several experimental conditions have been shown to trigger cell competition, including differential levels in ribosomal activity or in signalling pathway activation between cells, although it is unclear how those differences are sensed and translated into fitness levels. Many of the pathways implicated in cell competition have been previously linked with cancer, and this has led to the hypothesis that cell competition could play a role in tumour formation. Cell competition could be co-opted by cancer cells to kill surrounding normal cells and boost their own tissue colonization. However, in some cases, cell competition could have a tumour suppressor role, as cells harbouring mutations in a subset of tumour suppressor genes are killed by wild-type

[1]These authors contributed equally to this chapter.
[2]To whom correspondence should be addressed (email e.piddini@gurdon.cam.ac.uk).

cells. Originally described in developing epithelia, competitive interactions have also been observed in some stem cell niches, where they play a role in regulating stem cell selection, maintenance and tissue repopulation. Thus competitive interactions could be relevant to the maintenance of tissue fitness and have a protective role against aging.

Introduction

Cell competition occurs when cells with different fitness levels confront one another. It results in the elimination of the weaker population through apoptosis or senescence, whereas the stronger population survives and proliferates. Originally described in developing epithelia, competitive interactions have been linked with tissue homoeostasis, organ size control and stem cell maintenance. Recent work also suggests that they may play a role in tissue regeneration and in cancer development. In the present chapter we will introduce the pathways implicated in initiating competition and report on our current understanding of the mechanisms involved in this process.

Pathways of cell competition

Cell competition was discovered in 1975, through characterization of the growth defects of *Minute* heterozygous mutations in *Drosophila* wing imaginal discs [1]. *Minute* (*M*) genes encode ribosomal subunits. Thus homozygous mutations are lethal due to a lack of functional ribosomes; however, heterozygous animals are viable and display just a developmental delay and minor morphological abnormalities. These early studies from Morata, Ripoll and Simpson [1–3] showed that when *Minute* heterozygous (*M*/ +) and wild-type cells were present in the same tissue, wild-type cells would take over, whereas slow-growing *M*/ + cells were eliminated and their contribution to the adult wing was reduced. This suggested that competition could act as a surveillance system to actively remove mutant defective cells from the tissue. In 2004, Oliver et al. [4] reproduced these findings in a mouse *Minute* mutation (Belly Spot and Tail), providing the first indication that the phenomenon of cell competition seen in *Drosophila* also occurs in mice.

Over 20 years after these first observations were made, Johnston et al. [5] reported that cells with differing levels of the transcription factor dMyc could also initiate competition. Cells with low levels of dMyc, because of a mutation in the corresponding gene, were lost in the presence of wild-type cells, but were viable when surrounded by the same cells. Moreno and Basler [6] and de la Cova et al. [7] later showed that mutant clones overexpressing dMyc could outcompete wild-type cells, suggesting that it was the relative levels of dMyc that decided the outcome of competition. In other words, the outcome of competition is context-dependent and cells become winners or losers depending on the fitness of their neighbours. This work confirmed the concept of supercompetitors: cells capable of outcompeting normal wild-type cells [8]. The discovery of supercompetitors established the initial link between cell competition and cancer. The human homologue of *dmyc* is an established proto-oncogene, controlling the expression of many other genes involved in growth and proliferation and is frequently overexpressed in tumours [9]. Thus it was proposed that, similarly to what had been observed in *Drosophila*, cancer cells with high Myc levels could cause the elimination of surrounding normal cells, creating space in which to expand.

This view was further strengthened when mutations in tumour suppressors also gave rise to supercompetitors. The Hippo pathway modulates cell survival and proliferation and thus safeguards against neoplastic growth. Inactivation of this pathway through *yorkie* overexpression or mutations in *fat, expanded* or *warts* enables cells to eliminate surrounding wild-type tissue [10,11]. Similarly, Vincent et al. [12] showed that, in *Drosophila,* relative differences in Wnt signalling induce competition. In this study, cells that cannot transduce the Wnt signal or cells that overactivate the pathway (*APC* or *Axin* mutant) were juxtaposed to wild-type cells. In both cases, those cells with relatively lower Wnt signalling levels were eliminated. Wnt signalling is overactivated in a number of cancers and *Axin* and *APC* are frequently mutated tumour suppressor genes [13]. Thus cell competition could also play a role in Wnt-induced cancers.

Tumour-suppressor-based mechanisms of cell competition have also been studied *in vivo* in a mammalian system. The transcription factor p53 is one of the best-known and most studied tumour suppressor genes [14]. Bondar and Medzhitov [15] characterized a form of cell competition induced by stress and mediated by p53. Doing repopulation assays in lethally irradiated bone marrow, they found that in the mouse haemopoietic stem cell, niche cell competition selects for the least damaged cells by comparing levels of p53 activity and selecting those cells with relatively lower p53 levels. This work, carried out with mouse HSPCs (haemopoietic stem and progenitor cells), shows that competition is not restricted to epithelial tissues. In addition to this study, the occurrence of cell competition in stem cell niches has also been reported in the *Drosophila* ovary and testis [16–19]. Moreover, cell competition has been shown during liver repopulation assays in rats [20].

The above tumour suppressor mutations induce a supercompetitive behaviour; however, this is not always the case, loss-of-function of the tumour suppressor genes *scrib (scribble)* or *lgl (lethal giant larvae)* leads to their elimination by the surrounding wild-type cells, both in *Drosophila* mosaic discs and mammalian cells [21–24]. Thus not all tumour-promoting mutations lead to a competitive advantage, and in some cases precancerous cells can be eliminated by cell competition. How do mutations alter the competitive status of a cell and what cellular events take place during competition? We review the current knowledge in the following sections.

Sensing cellular fitness

By far the most mysterious aspect of the cell competition process is to understand how cells sense and compare fitness levels across tissues. What are the signals and mechanisms that cells use to compare fitness and how are less fit cells identified and earmarked as losers?

Several studies have highlighted a correlation between differential proliferation rates and cell competition. For example, slow-growing *Minute* cells behave as losers next to normally growing wild-type cells; in turn, wild-type cells behave as losers next to cells that grow faster, e.g. because of high Myc activity [1–3,6,7]. Thus it has been suggested that, during competition, information about growth rates is translated into fitness levels and accounts for the acquisition of the loser/winner status. However, not all manipulations that increase growth rates appear to be sufficient to change the competitive status of a cell. For example boosting cellular growth by overactivating the insulin pathway is not sufficient to induce a super-competitor status [7]. Therefore it is possible that cells do not compare growth rates; rather they sense differences in a parameter, whose changes mirror differences in growth rates in some instances.

Another clue in understanding how cells sense relative fitness levels comes from the many reports indicating that disparities in some signalling pathways often lead to cell competition. This has been described for the Fat/Hippo [11,22,25] and Wnt signalling pathways [12]. In addition it has been reported that, during *Minute* competition, loser cells display reduced Dpp [*Drosophila* TGF-β (transforming growth factor β) superfamily member] signalling and that increasing the levels of signalling is sufficient to rescue them during both *Minute*- and Myc-induced competition [6,26]; however, this view has been questioned in subsequent work [7,10,27]. Thus, although it is unclear how signalling levels are translated into fitness levels, it appears that several signalling pathways are able to modulate the levels of cell fitness that are compared during cell competition.

A recent breakthrough in the study of cell competition has come from the identification of a trio of proteins as important components of the fitness-sensing process. Performing transcriptional profiling of competing cells, Moreno and co-workers [28] showed that three differently spliced isoforms of the *flower* gene become differentially expressed in several contexts where competition is induced: the Flower ^{ubi} isoform is down-regulated in loser cells, whereas two other Flower isoforms, Flower ^{LoseA} and Flower ^{LoseB}, are exclusively up-regulated in loser cells. Importantly, expression of either Flower ^{Lose} isoform is necessary and sufficient for the elimination of loser cells [28]. The mechanism of action of the Flower proteins and how they induce death in losers is entirely unknown at present. Flower has been described in another study as a calcium transporter [29]; however, it is unclear whether this function is required for its role in competition. Since they are transmembrane proteins, it is likely that Flower proteins are involved in extracellular recognition events between winners and losers. However, it is worth noting that, since Flower ^{Lose} isoforms are not present at the onset of competition and become expressed only as competition is triggered, additional molecules must be responsible for the early sensing events that lead to the differential expression of the Flower isoforms.

The identification of membrane proteins as integral components of the fitness-sensing process indicates that some aspects of cell competition require cell–cell contact [28]. Moreover, additional studies have shown that competitive interactions are observed at a short range (ranging from direct proximity [30] to a few cell diameters away [7]). However, independent experiments in cell culture show that cell competition can still happen if winner and loser cells share the same culture medium but are not allowed direct contact [31]. Therefore it is possible that multiple independent molecular pathways initiate competition and that some of those are mediated by soluble factors. The nature of these factors remains to be identified: they could be signalling proteins or by-products of cellular metabolism. Interestingly, in the context of competition induced by Wnt signalling, high-Wnt cells release Notum, a diffusible Wnt inhibitor that is required for the outcompetition of low-Wnt cells [12]. Notum does not take part in the fitness-sensing process, but contributes to competition by lowering the Wnt signalling levels (and hence fitness) of surrounding wild-type cells.

Elimination of loser cells

As described in the Introduction, a key feature of cell competition is the non-autonomous induction of death in the weaker population. How are loser cells instructed to die by neighbouring winner cells? With one exception, in which loser outcompetition happens via induction of senescence rather than death (discussed below), loser cells are killed by apoptosis (Figure 1). However, while this is a common denominator, several independent upstream pathways have been shown to trigger the apoptotic event during cell competition. Their involvement seems to be context-dependent and influenced by the specific type of cell competition studied and possibly by the tissue studied (Figure 1A).

Activation of the JNK (c-Jun N-terminal kinase) pathway, a pro-apoptotic pathway frequently activated in response to stress [32], is quite a common event during competition, having been observed during *Minute* [26] and Myc [6] competition (Figure 1A) and during competition induced by mutations in polarity-linked tumour suppressors [33,34]. Is JNK activation required to induce death in loser cells? With respect to *Minute* and Myc competition there is some controversy. Some studies report that blocking JNK in loser cells inhibits their apoptosis and rescues them from competition [6,26]; however, independent reports found that inactivating the JNK pathway had little or no effect on cell competition [7,10]. In the case of competition induced by mutations in polarity-linked tumour suppressors, the data instead rather unequivocally shows that JNK signalling plays a key role [22,34,35] (Figure 1B). In *scrib*$^{-/-}$ cells, altered endocytic trafficking leads to hyperactivation of Eiger [*Drosophila* TNF (tumour necrosis factor) superfamily member] signalling,

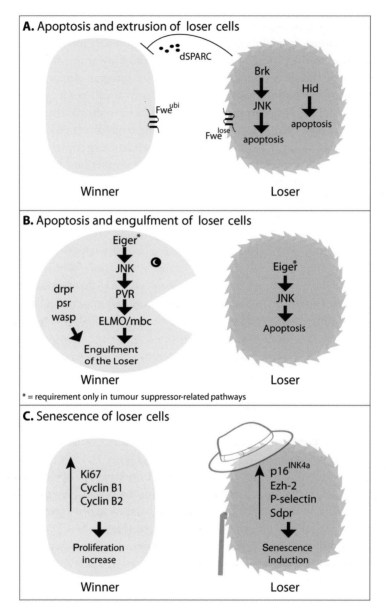

Figure 1. Mechanisms involved in the elimination of loser cells
(**A**) Apoptosis and extrusion of loser cells. Two mechanisms of apoptosis induction have been identified. In the first, JNK is activated via Brk (Brinker), whereas in the second activation of the pro-apototic gene *Hid* leads to death. Different Fwe (Flower) isoforms label winner and loser cells. dSPARC is secreted from loser cells and acts as a temporary shield to protect them from apoptosis. (**B**) Apoptosis and engulfment of loser cells. In some contexts, winner cells engulf neighbouring loser cells, via activation of genes involved in phagocytosis (listed in the Figure). This is regulated by Eiger/JNK activation, which promotes apoptosis in the losers and engulfment in the winners. (**C**) Senescence of loser cells. Competition among HSPCs results in the activation of senescence-related genes in the loser cells (listed in the Figure). Conversely, winner cells activate proliferation markers (listed in the Figure).

which results in JNK activation [34]. Importantly, in this context Eiger/JNK signalling has a dual function. In addition to being active within scrib[-/-] cells, where it promotes apoptosis, Eiger/JNK signalling becomes activated in a row of wild-type cells just surrounding the mutant scrib[-/-] tissue. There, JNK activation has quite the opposite effect, since it is required for these cells to eliminate their scrib[-/-] neighbours [33]. Interestingly, a recent study shows that, in a mammalian cell culture model of scrib cell competition, scrib[-/-] cells do not activate JNK, but activate p38 MAPK (mitogen-activated protein kinase), another kinase activated by cellular stress. In this context, p38 activation is required for the apoptosis of scrib[-/-] cells [36].

Interestingly, Eiger is not an obligate upstream activator of JNK during competition. For example, during *Minute* competition, Eiger function has no obvious effects on the elimination of *Minute* cells [33], whereas JNK inhibition rescues, at least partially, the outcompetition of loser cells [6,7]. This would suggest that Eiger is dispensable for JNK activation. Consistent with this, JNK activation during *Minute* competition requires Brinker, a transcriptional repressor that is up-regulated in competing *Minute* cells and also becomes required for their apoptosis [26].

As a consequence of cell competition a tissue may be presented with a substantial increase in the amount of apoptotic cells. What is the fate of such apoptotic bodies and how are they cleared from the tissue? Initial observations reported that, in wing imaginal discs apoptotic cells are extruded from the epithelial layer and accumulate basally [6] where they are probably cleared by macrophages. It was later found that during *Minute* and Myc competition, apoptotic bodies are engulfed by surrounding winner cells [30]. In other words, during competition fitter cells eat their less-fit neighbours (Figure 1B). This has also been observed recently for scrib[-/-] cells, which are engulfed by surrounding wild-type neighbours [33]. In both studies it was found that molecular components normally involved in phagocytosis are required for cell engulfment [30,33]. In a surprising turn, both studies further reported that cell engulfment is not simply a secondary event that clears cellular debris from the tissue; rather it is an active and essential component of the cell competition process. This conclusion is on the basis of the observation that inhibiting the function of proteins required for engulfment actually leads to inhibition of competition. Since both studies confirmed this finding by targeting several components of the phagocytic machinery, the evidence for a requirement of engulfment in competition is strong [30,33]; however alternative explanations are possible. For example, removing the function of these genes could reduce cellular fitness. Alternatively, mutations in these genes could affect endocytic trafficking, which has been shown to modulate cell competition [6,34].

Regardless of whether they are simply extruded or actively engulfed, loser cells do not die without putting up a fight. A recent report shows that, during the early stages of competition, loser cells express dSPARC (*Drosophila* secreted protein acidic and rich in cysteine) [37], a secreted matricellular glycoprotein involved in extracellular matrix remodelling and in modulating the activity of multiple signalling pathways [38]. dSPARC expression temporarily protects loser cells from competition by delaying the induction of apoptosis, although the exact mechanism is not presently understood. It is proposed that dSPARC acts as a shield to delay the effect of cell competition. This would avoid unnecessary elimination of cells that are able to recover from transient damage [37].

Recent work studying cell competition in the HSPC niche found that outcompeted cells may actually survive [15]. In this context, the outcome of cell competition is induction of senescence in outcompeted stem cells (Figure 1C). Gene expression profiling shows that, during competition, loser cells up-regulate the senescence-related genes $p16^{(INK4a)}$ and $Ezh-2$, and have high levels of P-$selectin$ and $Sdpr$, which are normally up-regulated in aged HSPCs [15]. Ultimately, since senescent cells are permanently cell-cycle-arrested, the outcome is not dissimilar from other modes of competition; although they remain alive, loser cells are inhibited from repopulating the niche.

Tissue colonization by winner cells

During cell competition, despite the intense elimination of loser cells, organ size and tissue growth are unaffected and overall cell number is conserved. This is possible because, as loser cells die, winner cells display a corresponding increase in the rate of proliferation. This has been observed during *Minute* competition [30] (although it has been questioned [27]) and in other competitive contexts. Thus high-Myc cells overproliferate as a consequence of competition [6,31] and HSPCs with relatively low levels of p53 up-regulate markers of cell proliferation under competitive conditions, such as *Ki67*, *cyclin B1* and *cyclin A2* [15] (Figure 1C). Thus cell competition can, at least in some cases, increase winner cell proliferation. Importantly, in one instance where this was investigated, growth stimulation appeared to be induced at a short-range. Elegant genetic experiments conducted by Simpson and Morata [3] showed that, during *Minute* competition, clones of winner cells display increased growth if they are in the proximity of loser cells, but not if they are further away from the site of competition. However, in *Drosophila* cell culture models of competition, where cell–cell contact is not required for apoptosis induction, winner cell overproliferation is also triggered in the absence of cell contact [31].

Cell competition and disease

A quality-control mechanism
Cell-autonomous apoptosis is activated in cells that sustain major functional damage, but how are viable, but suboptimal, cells removed? During development, cell competition acts as a quality-control mechanism that eliminates suboptimal cells before they contribute to the adult organism (Figure 2A). Is there also a role for cell competition in maintaining organ fitness in the adult? Adult

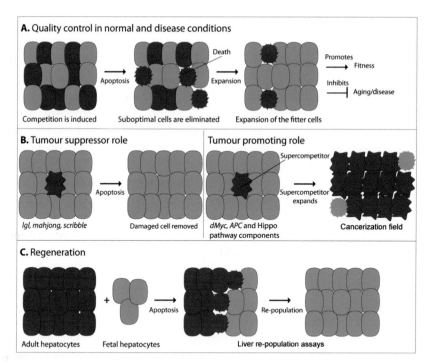

Figure 2. Potential links between cell competition and disease

(**A**) Quality control in normal and disease conditions. Suboptimal cells are eliminated from epithelial tissues through apoptosis, whereas the fitter cells show a corresponding increase in proliferation. (**B**) Tumour suppressor role. Cell competition could act as a protective mechanism to remove potentially dangerous cells from a tissue, thus preventing tumour formation. Tumour promoting role. By contrast, cell competition could be exploited by mutant cells to promote tumour formation. Mutant supercompetitor cells with precancerous lesions could outcompete and cull surrounding wild-type cells, leading to the generation of cancerization fields. (**C**) Regeneration. On the basis of experiments in liver repopulation assays, it has been proposed that cell competition could be exploited in regenerative medicine.

tissues, as a consequence of environmental stress or damage, accumulate suboptimal cells. One way to neutralize them is through the induction of cellular senescence, which leads to a permanent cell proliferation arrest [39]. However, this appears not to be ideal, as a recent study shows that the accumulation of senescent cells during aging contributes to the insurgence of age-related pathologies [40]. Thus it could be proposed that cell competition eliminates damaged cells before the activation of senescence. By selecting fitter cells and reducing the number of senescent cells, cell competition could contribute to maintaining organ fitness and delaying tissue aging. However, a recent study indicates that cell competition itself could lead to the accumulation of senescent cells in HSPCs [15]. This could be a peculiarity of the HSPC niche. In addition, it is unclear whether in this system a proportion of loser cells are also eliminated by cell death during competition.

Cell competition could be relevant to a number of human diseases. In a rare sporadic skin disorder (ichthyosis with confetti) it is observed that patients develop patches of healthy skin within abnormal skin areas [41]. Each patch originates from clonal expansion of a single revertant stem cell which has lost the dominant mutation in *keratin-10*. In some patients more than a thousand revertant clones are seen, suggesting that these stem cells produce healthy skin cells able to outcompete surrounding diseased tissue. Competition could also be involved in non-random X-chromosome inactivation, seen in various X-linked immunodeficiencies [42]. In female mammals random inactivation of one of the two X-chromosomes occurs in every somatic cell during early development. Once X-inactivation has taken place all clonal descendents will have the same X inactivated. In a number of X-linked genetic diseases, preferential tissue-specific inactivation of one X-chromosome is seen. In these contexts, cells inactivating the mutant allele could gain an advantage over cells in which the normal allele is inactivated. Although not proven, removal of mutated cells could be occurring via a mechanism similar to cell competition.

Cancer

Cell competition has been linked to cancer, as many of the genes involved are also known vertebrate oncogenes or tumour suppressors. Initially cell competition was thought of as a mechanism that would favour the growth of tumour cells [6]. The discovery of genes which could transform cells into supercompetitors led to the hypothesis that cells with precancerous lesions could over-colonize the tissue by eliminating the surrounding cells (Figure 2B) [6–8,11]. This expanded population of cells would then be more likely to undergo further mutations, finally allowing the cells to overcome the restraints of the tissue and develop into a tumour. This theory is consistent with the model of field cancerization, which was proposed to explain the development of multiple concomitant primary tumours in the same tissue, together with the observation that abnormal tissue often surrounds the tumour [43,44]. It was thus proposed that early precancerous lesions could allow cells to expand and colonize the tissue. In this field, further independent genetic hits at multiple tissue locations would give rise to tumours that share a monoclonal origin [43,44]. This model is indeed supported by the fact that tumour-associated genetic mutations are frequently present in biopsies taken from the macroscopically normal mucosa adjacent to the tumour [43,44]. Competition could also be involved in helping tumour cells establish themselves at secondary sites during formation of metastasis.

More recently it has been shown that cell competition could also play an opposite role during cancer formation. In fact there are now observations suggesting that surrounding normal cells can suppress the proliferation of tumour cells. Cells mutated in the tumour suppressors *scrib* and *lgl* are eliminated by wild-type cells, indicating that cell competition could act as a tumour suppressor mechanism eliminating potentially harmful cells from the tissue [21–24].

Manipulating cell competition during cancer formation could provide an alternative new strategy to fight cancer. The emergence of new *in vitro* cell culture competition assays means it is now possible to study competition between normal and transformed cells in mammalian systems [35]. The discovery of competition-specific genes will be essential in establishing these new therapies and in identifying novel biomarkers for early detection.

Tissue regeneration

The established role of cell competition in controlling cell proliferation suggests that competition could be relevant for regenerative medicine (Figure 2C). In 2006 Oertel et al. [20] demonstrated that the process of cell competition could be used to replace functional tissue in the adult liver by fetal liver progenitors. They observed that younger highly proliferative fetal cells replaced slower growing adult cells by inducing apoptosis. This strategy could serve to design effective treatments of regenerative medicine for a wide variety of disorders.

Conclusions

Since the original discovery of cell competition over 35 years ago, the field has made tremendous advances. In particular, the list of experimental conditions that trigger cell competition continues to grow, suggesting that this is a frequently occurring phenomenon. Most importantly, there is now ample evidence that this is also a mammalian event. However, several unanswered questions remain. Although some progress has been made, the molecular mechanisms of cell competition are still largely unknown. Furthermore, we are still to fully grasp its physiological relevance in health and disease, and to realise its potential for biomedical applications. The next decade will undoubtedly be an exciting time for this field of research.

Summary

- *Many experimental conditions have been shown to result in cell competition, including defects in ribosomal proteins and alterations in growth factor signalling levels. It is likely that multiple independent pathways initiate competition.*
- *Differences in cellular fitness may be induced by differential growth rates, signalling pathway levels or expression of extracellular proteins.*
- *Loser cells are eliminated through apoptosis or senescence. Several independent pathways trigger these events depending on the context of competition.*
- *Outcompeted loser cells can be expelled from epithelial tissues through extrusion or active engulfment.*
- *Organ growth and tissue size are maintained during competition: as loser cells die the winners show a corresponding increase in proliferation.*
- *Cell competition acts as a quality-control mechanism to eliminate suboptimal cells during development and possibly also in the adult.*

- *Cell competition has been implicated in liver repopulation assays and it has been proposed that it could therefore be used in regenerative medicine.*

References

1. Morata, G. and Ripoll, P. (1975) Minutes: mutants of *Drosophila* autonomously affecting cell division rate. Dev. Biol. **42**, 211–221
2. Simpson, P. (1979) Parameters of cell competition in the compartments of the wing disc of *Drosophila*. Dev. Biol. **69**, 182–193
3. Simpson, P. and Morata, G. (1981) Differential mitotic rates and patterns of growth in compartments in the *Drosophila* wing. Dev. Biol. **85**, 299–308
4. Oliver, E.R., Saunders, T.L., Tarle, S.A. and Glaser, T. (2004) Ribosomal protein L24 defect in belly spot and tail (Bst), a mouse Minute. Development **131**, 3907–3920
5. Johnston, L.A., Prober, D.A., Edgar, B.A., Eisenman, R.N. and Gallant, P. (1999) *Drosophila* myc regulates cellular growth during development. Cell **98**, 779–790
6. Moreno, E. and Basler, K. (2004) dMyc transforms cells into super-competitors. Cell **117**, 117–129
7. de la Cova, C., Abril, M., Bellosta, P., Gallant, P. and Johnston, L.A. (2004) *Drosophila* myc regulates organ size by inducing cell competition. Cell **117**, 107–116
8. Abrams, J.M. (2002) Competition and compensation: coupled to death in development and cancer. Cell **110**, 403–406
9. Donaldson, T.D. and Duronio, R.J. (2004) Cancer cell biology: Myc wins the competition. Curr. Biol. **14**, R425–R427
10. Tyler, D.M., Li, W., Zhuo, N., Pellock, B. and Baker, N.E. (2007) Genes affecting cell competition in *Drosophila*. Genetics **175**, 643–657
11. Ziosi, M., Baena-Lopez, L.A., Grifoni, D., Froldi, F., Pession, A., Garoia, F., Trotta, V., Bellosta, P. and Cavicchi, S. (2010) dMyc functions downstream of Yorkie to promote the supercompetitive behavior of hippo pathway mutant cells. PLoS Genet. **6**, e1001140
12. Vincent, J.P., Kolahgar, G., Gagliardi, M. and Piddini, E. (2011) Steep differences in wingless signaling trigger Myc-independent competitive cell interactions. Dev. Cell **21**, 366–374
13. Polakis, P. (2000) Wnt signaling and cancer. Genes Dev. **14**, 1837–1851
14. Vazquez, A., Bond, E.E., Levine, A.J. and Bond, G.L. (2008) The genetics of the p53 pathway, apoptosis and cancer therapy. Nat. Rev. Drug Discovery **7**, 979–987
15. Bondar, T. and Medzhitov, R. (2010) p53-mediated hematopoietic stem and progenitor cell competition. Cell Stem Cell **6**, 309–322
16. Rhiner, C., Diaz, B., Portela, M., Poyatos, J.F., Fernandez-Ruiz, I., Lopez-Gay, J.M., Gerlitz, O. and Moreno, E. (2009) Persistent competition among stem cells and their daughters in the *Drosophila* ovary germline niche. Development **136**, 995–1006
17. Issigonis, M., Tulina, N., de Cuevas, M., Brawley, C., Sandler, L. and Matunis, E. (2009) JAK-STAT signal inhibition regulates competition in the *Drosophila* testis stem cell niche. Science **326**, 153–156
18. Jin, Z., Kirilly, D., Weng, C., Kawase, E., Song, X., Smith, S., Schwartz, J. and Xie, T. (2008) Differentiation-defective stem cells outcompete normal stem cells for niche occupancy in the *Drosophila* ovary. Cell Stem Cell **2**, 39–49
19. Sheng, X.R., Brawley, C.M. and Matunis, E.L. (2009) Dedifferentiating spermatogonia outcompete somatic stem cells for niche occupancy in the *Drosophila* testis. Cell Stem Cell **5**, 191–203
20. Oertel, M., Menthena, A., Dabeva, M.D. and Shafritz, D.A. (2006) Cell competition leads to a high level of normal liver reconstitution by transplanted fetal liver stem/progenitor cells. Gastroenterology **130**, 507–520

21. Brumby, A.M. and Richardson, H.E. (2003) Scribble mutants cooperate with oncogenic Ras or Notch to cause neoplastic overgrowth in *Drosophila*. EMBO J. **22**, 5769–5779

22. Menendez, J., Perez-Garijo, A., Calleja, M. and Morata, G. (2010) A tumor-suppressing mechanism in *Drosophila* involving cell competition and the Hippo pathway. Proc. Natl. Acad. Sci. U.S.A **107**, 14651–14656

23. Grzeschik, N.A., Amin, N., Secombe, J., Brumby, A.M. and Richardson, H.E. (2007) Abnormalities in cell proliferation and apico-basal cell polarity are separable in *Drosophila* lgl mutant clones in the developing eye. Dev. Biol. **311**, 106–123

24. Froldi, F., Ziosi, M., Garoia, F., Pession, A., Grzeschik, N.A., Bellosta, P., Strand, D., Richardson, H.E. and Grifoni, D. (2010) The lethal giant larvae tumour suppressor mutation requires dMyc oncoprotein to promote clonal malignancy. BMC Biol. **8**, 33

25. Neto-Silva, R.M., de Beco, S. and Johnston, L.A. (2010) Evidence for a growth-stabilizing regulatory feedback mechanism between Myc and Yorkie, the *Drosophila* homolog of Yap. Dev. Cell **19**, 507–520

26. Moreno, E., Basler, K. and Morata, G. (2002) Cells compete for decapentaplegic survival factor to prevent apoptosis in *Drosophila* wing development. Nature **416**, 755–759

27. Martin, F.A., Herrera, S.C. and Morata, G. (2009) Cell competition, growth and size control in the *Drosophila* wing imaginal disc. Development **136**, 3747–3756

28. Rhiner, C., Lopez-Gay, J.M., Soldini, D., Casas-Tinto, S., Martin, F.A., Lombardia, L. and Moreno, E. (2010) Flower forms an extracellular code that reveals the fitness of a cell to its neighbors in *Drosophila*. Dev. Cell **18**, 985–998

29. Yao, C.K., Lin, Y.Q., Ly, C.V., Ohyama, T., Haueter, C. M., Moiseenkova-Bell, V.Y., Wensel, T.G. and Bellen, H.J. (2009) A synaptic vesicle-associated Ca^{2+} channel promotes endocytosis and couples exocytosis to endocytosis. Cell **138**, 947–960

30. Li, W. and Baker, N.E. (2007) Engulfment is required for cell competition. Cell **129**, 1215–1225

31. Senoo-Matsuda, N. and Johnston, L.A. (2007) Soluble factors mediate competitive and cooperative interactions between cells expressing different levels of *Drosophila* Myc. Proc. Natl. Acad. Sci. U.S.A. **104**, 18543–18548

32. Bogoyevitch, M.A. and Kobe, B. (2006) Uses for JNK: the many and varied substrates of the c-Jun N-terminal kinases. Microbiol. Mol. Biol. Rev. **70**, 1061–1095

33. Ohsawa, S., Sugimura, K., Takino, K., Xu, T., Miyawaki, A. and Igaki, T. (2011) Elimination of oncogenic neighbors by JNK-mediated engulfment in *Drosophila*. Dev. Cell **20**, 315–328

34. Igaki, T., Pastor-Pareja, J.C., Aonuma, H., Miura, M. and Xu, T. (2009) Intrinsic tumor suppression and epithelial maintenance by endocytic activation of Eiger/TNF signaling in *Drosophila*. Dev. Cell **16**, 458–465

35. Tamori, Y., Bialucha, C.U., Tian, A.G., Kajita, M., Huang, Y.C., Norman, M., Harrison, N., Poulton, J., Ivanovitch, K., Disch, L. et al. (2010) Involvement of Lgl and Mahjong/VprBP in cell competition. PLoS Biol. **8**, e1000422

36. Norman, M., Wisniewska, K.A., Lawrenson, K., Garcia-Miranda, P., Tada, M., Kajita, M., Mano, H., Ishikawa, S., Ikegawa, M., Shimada, T. and Fujita, Y. (2012) Loss of Scribble causes cell competition in mammalian cells. J. Cell Sci. **125**, 59–66

37. Portela, M., Casas-Tinto, S., Rhiner, C., Lopez-Gay, J. M., Dominguez, O., Soldini, D. and Moreno, E. (2010) *Drosophila* SPARC is a self-protective signal expressed by loser cells during cell competition. Dev. Cell **19**, 562–573

38. Clark, C.J. and Sage, E.H. (2008) A prototypic matricellular protein in the tumor microenvironment: where there's SPARC, there's fire. J. Cell. Biochem. **104**, 721–732

39. Kuilman, T., Michaloglou, C., Mooi, W. J. and Peeper, D.S. (2010) The essence of senescence. Genes Dev. **24**, 2463–2479

40. Baker, D.J., Wijshake, T., Tchkonia, T., LeBrasseur, N.K., Childs, B.G., van de Sluis, B., Kirkland, J.L. and van Deursen, J.M. (2011) Clearance of p16Ink4a-positive senescent cells delays ageing-associated disorders. Nature **479**, 232–236

41.   Choate, K.A., Lu, Y., Zhou, J., Choi, M., Elias, P.M., Farhi, A., Nelson-Williams, C., Crumrine, D., Williams, M.L., Nopper, A.J. et al. (2010) Mitotic recombination in patients with ichthyosis causes reversion of dominant mutations in KRT10. Science **330**, 94–97

42.   Puck, J.M., Stewart, C.C. and Nussbaum, R.L. (1992) Maximum-likelihood analysis of human T-cell X chromosome inactivation patterns: normal women versus carriers of X-linked severe combined immunodeficiency. Am. J. Hum. Genet. **50**, 742–748

43.   Slaughter, D.P., Southwick, H.W. and Smejkal, W. (1953) Field cancerization in oral stratified squamous epithelium; clinical implications of multicentric origin. Cancer **6**, 963–968

44.   Braakhuis, B.J., Tabor, M.P., Kummer, J.A., Leemans, C.R. and Brakenhoff, R.H. (2003) A genetic explanation of Slaughter's concept of field cancerization: evidence and clinical implications. Cancer Res. **63**, 1727–1730

© The Authors Journal compilation © 2012 Biochemical Society
Essays Biochem. (2012) **53**, 83–93: doi: 10.1042/BSE0530083

7

The control of gene expression and cell proliferation by the epithelial apical junctional complex

Domenica Spadaro*†, Rocio Tapia*†, Pamela Pulimeno† and Sandra Citi*†1

Department of Cell Biology, University of Geneva, 4 Boulevard d'Yvoy, CH-1211-4 Geneva, Switzerland, and †Department of Molecular Biology, University of Geneva, 4 Boulevard d'Yvoy, CH-1211-4 Geneva, Switzerland

Abstract

The AJC (apical junctional complex) of vertebrate epithelial cells orchestrates cell–cell adhesion and tissue barrier function. In addition, it plays a pivotal role in signalling. Several protein components of the AJC, e.g. the cytoplasmic proteins β-catenin, p120-catenin and ZO (Zonula Occludens)-2, can shuttle to the nucleus, where they interact with transcription factors to regulate gene expression and cell proliferation. Other junctional proteins, e.g. angiomotin, α-catenin and cingulin, are believed to act by sequestering either transcription factors, such as YAP (Yes-associated protein), or regulators of small GTPases, such as GEF (guanine-nucleotide-exchange factor)-H1, at junctions. The signalling activities of AJC proteins are triggered by different extracellular and intracellular cues, including cell density, and physiological or pathological activation of developmentally regulated pathways, such as the Wnt pathway. The interplay between

¹To whom correspondence should be addressed (email Sandra.Citi@unige.ch).

junctional protein complexes, the actin cytoskeleton and signalling pathways is of crucial importance in the regulation of gene expression and cell proliferation.

Introduction

Epithelial proliferation and gene expression must be tightly controlled during development and in adult tissues, and are dysregulated in cancer. In the present chapter, we review recent advances in understanding the role of cell–cell junctions, and specifically the AJC (apical junctional complex), in the regulation of cell proliferation and gene expression in vertebrate epithelial cells.

The AJC comprises the ZO (Zonula Occludens) [TJ (tight junction)] and the zonula adherens [AJ (adherens junction)]. Each of these junctions consists of a multi-molecular complex of transmembrane and cytoplasmic proteins, which are linked to the cytoskeleton. Claudins, occludin, tricellulin and JAM-A (junctional adhesion molecule A), and E-cadherin and nectin are the major transmembrane proteins of TJs and AJs respectively [1,2]. The cytoplasmic domains of TJ membrane proteins interact with scaffolding proteins (ZO-1, ZO-2, ZO-3 and others) and directly or indirectly with polarity complex proteins [PAR-3, PAR-6 and others (PAR is PARtioning defective)]. The cytoplasmic tail of E-cadherin interacts with β-catenin and p120-ctn (p120-catenin), whereas nectin binds to the afadin–ponsin complex. TJs and AJs contain several other proteins which serve as adaptors for signalling molecules, and provide linkages to the actin and microtubule cytoskeletons [1–3]. The cytoskeleton functions as a structural organizer of junctions and polarity, and induces cell shape changes through the development of tensile strength and its regulated assembly.

The functions of the AJC are critical in the development and physiology of vertebrate organisms. The TJ provides epithelial tissues with a semi-permeable barrier to the passage of solutes through the paracellular pathway, and contribute to maintaining apical–basal polarity [2,3]. The neighbouring AJ plays a fundamental role in initiating and maintaining cell–cell adhesion [1]. However, besides these canonical functions, exciting new roles for TJs and AJs in signalling have been discovered in the last two decades. In this chapter, we describe the major proteins and mechanisms that are involved in the control of gene expression and cell proliferation by the AJC. The reader should be aware that the field is considerably more complex than presented here, and is referred to a review [4] for a more complete introduction to this field.

AJ proteins and nucleo-cytoplasmic signalling

The AJ proteins p120-ctn and β-catenin not only modulate the stability of E-cadherin and its interaction with the actin and microtubule cytoskeletons [1], but also have crucial signalling functions. Both proteins show a nuclear localization in proliferating cells, and interact with and tune the activity of transcription factors. A third catenin, α-catenin, associates with E-cadherin by binding to β-catenin, and

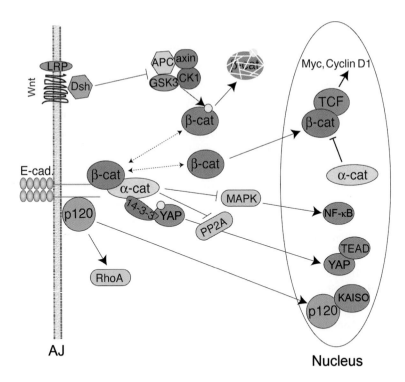

Figure 1. Regulation of signalling by AJs
The junctional membrane and the nucleus are schematically represented on the left and the right respectively. For simplicity, only E-cadherin is shown as a transmembrane adhesion receptor of the AJ, and many other proteins are left out of this scheme. Only selected proteins and complexes are shown, and their interactions are indicated by lines and arrows. Phosphorylation is indicated by a yellow circle. The degradation of β-catenin (β-cat) is inhibited by the Wnt-dependent inhibition of the destruction complex, and free β-catenin migrates to the nucleus. α-Catenin (α-cat) controls proliferation of keratinocytes through inhibition of MAPK signalling, and by inhibiting PP2A, thus promoting the cytoplasmic retention of phosphorylated YAP. Both β-catenin and p120-ctn (p120) bind to transcription factors (TCF and KAISO respectively) in the nucleus. See the text for additional details. Dsh, Dishevelled.

has also been implicated in the control of gene expression and in the regulation of the nucleo-cytoplasmic shuttling of transcription factors (Figure 1).

Studies in *Drosophila* were the first to show that armadillo, the fly β-catenin homologue, is a downstream target of the Wnt signalling pathway. In the absence of Wnt ligand, β-catenin is bound to cadherin, and the free cytoplasmic β-catenin is rapidly degraded via phosphorylation by a destruction complex, which includes two scaffolding proteins, axin and APC (adenomatous polyposis coli), and two kinases, GSK (glycogen synthase kinase) 3β and CK1 (casein kinase 1) (Figure 1). The phosphorylated β-catenin is ubiquitinated, and then degraded by the proteasome. The interaction between the Wnt ligand and its receptors [frizzled and LRP (low-density-lipoprotein-receptor-related protein)] (Figure 1) inactivates the destruction complex and, consequently, β-catenin is not phosphorylated and accumulates in the cytoplasm. The stable cytoplasmic β-catenin translocates into the nucleus, where it acts as a co-activator of the transcription factor TCF (T-cell factor) to promote the expression of Wnt target genes [5], which include Myc and cyclin D1 (Figure 1). Wnt target genes in turn promote cell proliferation in developing tissues, and are important for the maintenance of stem cell properties in regenerating adult tissues. Significantly, many types of cancers are associated with mutations that lead to a pathological hyperactivation of the Wnt pathway. Wnt signalling is modulated not only by β-catenin, but also by other catenins. For example, α-catenin can negatively regulate β-catenin signalling, either by sequestering β-catenin in the cytoplasm or by inhibiting the β-catenin interaction with TCF (Figure 1).

p120-ctn and α-catenin regulate nuclear signalling and proliferation through additional Wnt-independent mechanisms. p120-ctn shuttles to the nucleus, although it is not clear whether this depends on its phosphorylation state, like β-catenin, or is regulated by the levels of E-cadherin, which recruits p120-ctn to junctions. In the nucleus, p120-ctn interacts with the repressor KAISO, leading to dissociation of KAISO from DNA, and transcription of KAISO target genes [6], which also include some Wnt target genes (Figure 1). α-Catenin acts as a tumour suppressor, since its conditional ablation in the epidermis induces hyperproliferation, activation of the Ras-MAPK (mitogen-activated protein kinase) pathway, and activation of NF-κB (nuclear factor κB) and its pro-inflammatory target genes [7] (Figure 1). Recently, it has been shown that α-catenin controls the nucleo-cytoplasmic shuttling of the transcription factor YAP (Yes-associated protein), an effector of the Hippo pathway [8,9] (see also the section on YAP below).

The role of ZO proteins, symplekin and ZONAB (ZO-1-associated nucleic acid-binding protein) in the control of gene expression and cell proliferation

The ZO proteins (ZO-1, ZO-2 and ZO-3) are essential cytoplasmic components of TJs (Figure 2), since they form scaffolds to anchor TJ membrane proteins, and link them to actin filaments [2]. However, they also play very important roles in signalling and in the control of gene expression and cell proliferation [4].

Some of the first evidence that ZO proteins were implicated in the control of gene expression was the observation that ZO-1 forms a complex with the transcription factor ZONAB, and that ZO-1 overexpression modulates the ZONAB-dependent transcription of the gene Erb-B2 [10] (Figure 2). ZONAB is localized at TJs in confluent cells, in a complex with CDK4 (cyclin-dependent kinase 4), but it translocates to the nucleus in sparse proliferating cells [10,11] (Figure 2). Nuclear translocation of ZONAB results in increased expression of genes involved in cell proliferation, such as cyclin D1 and PCNA (proliferation cell nuclear antigen) (Figure 2). ZONAB also functionally interacts with symplekin [12], a RNA-processing factor that shuttles between the TJ and the nucleus, where it interacts with the transcription factor HSF1 (heat-shock factor protein 1) to regulate the polyadenylation of Hsp70 (heat-shock protein 70) mRNA [13] (Figure 2). The

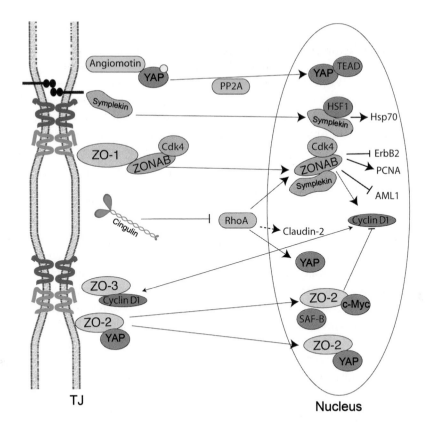

Figure 2. Regulation of signalling by TJs
The junctional membrane and the nucleus are schematically represented on the left and the right respectively. The TJ transmembrane proteins which are schematically depicted here are (from top to bottom) JAM, claudins and occludin. Only the major cytoplasmic TJ proteins that have been implicated in the control of gene expression, cell proliferation and localization of transcription factors are shown. The genes whose expression is modulated by the different proteins are indicated by text, except for cyclin D1, which is associated with ZO-3 at junctions during mitosis. Functional interactions and nuclear shuttling are indicated by arrows and lines. See the text for additional details.

symplekin–ZONAB complex has multiple targets and, in intestinal cells, it inhibits cell differentiation by repressing the transcription factor AML1 (acute myeloid leukaemia 1) [14] (Figure 2).

ZO-2 is the only ZO protein that has unequivocally been shown to translocate to the nucleus. ZO-2 binds to the transcription factor c-Myc, thus inhibiting the transcription, translation and degradation of cyclin D1, and consequently blocking cell-cycle progression at G_0/G_1 [15] (Figure 2). In addition, ZO-2 interacts with other transcription factors, including Jun/Fos and the scaffold attachment factor SAF-B, with as yet unknown effects [16,17] (Figure 2).

Unlike ZO-1 and ZO-2, the third ZO protein, ZO-3, appears to promote cell proliferation, since it recruits cyclin D1 to TJs during mitosis in intestinal cells, thus preventing its degradation, and thus promoting cell-cycle progression through S-phase [18]. The junctional recruitment of cyclin D1 requires a conserved sequence motif, which mediates interaction with PDZ [PSD-95 (post-synaptic density 95), Dlg (discs large) and ZO-1] domains [18]. PDZ domains are evolutionarily conserved protein modules, which mediate protein–protein interactions, and are found not only in ZO proteins, but in several other scaffolding proteins of TJs. Recruitment of transcription factors and signalling molecules to junctions through PDZ proteins might therefore be a general mechanism to control their subcellular localization and stability.

YAP, a regulator of cell growth, is controlled by junctional proteins

In mammals, cell and organ growth and size are regulated by organ-extrinsic factors, such as nutrition, growth factors and hormones, and by organ-intrinsic mechanisms. The Hippo pathway, which was originally described in *Drosophila*, is an organ-intrinsic mechanism, which acts by controlling two opposite processes: cell proliferation and apoptosis (see also Chapter 9 in this volume). The Hippo pathway consists of a cascade of kinases, which ultimately phosphorylate downstream effectors, such as the transcription factors YAP and its paralogue TAZ (transcriptional coactivator with PDZ-binding motif). When YAP and TAZ are not phosphorylated, they migrate into the nucleus, interact with the transcription factor TEAD, and promote the expression of proliferation-associated genes. When they are phosphorylated by the Hippo pathway kinases MST [mammalian Ste20 (sterile 20)-like kinase] 1/2 and LATS (large tumour suppressor), YAP and TAZ remain in the cytoplasm and either interact with proteins such as 14-3-3 (Figure 1) or are degraded (see also Chapter 9 in this volume).

Very importantly, experiments by different laboratories have highlighted a role for junctional proteins as upstream regulators of YAP localization. First, AMOT (angiomotin), a protein localized in the cytoplasmic domain of TJs, modulates the Hippo signalling pathway by interacting with YAP and its related protein TAZ [19,20] (Figure 2). AMOT recruits YAP to TJs, and stabilizes the phosphorylated form of YAP, thus inhibiting its nuclear translocation (Figure 2). Interestingly, the YAP paralogue TAZ interacts with the basal polarity complex protein Scribble to regulate cancer stem-cell related traits [21].

Another cytoplasmic TJ protein, ZO-2, interacts with YAP, and has been implicated in driving YAP to the nucleus, independently of phosphorylation [22] (Figure 2). Moreover, the AJ protein α-catenin is a major regulator of YAP localization and activity in the skin. In basal keratinocytes and stem cells of hair follicles α-catenin interacts with YAP through the 14-3-3 protein (Figure 1), and the loss of α-catenin leads to a nuclear re-localization of YAP, together with an increase in cell proliferation and tumour progression [8,9]. α-Catenin helps to maintain the phosphorylated state of YAP by preventing its association with the phosphatase PP2A (protein phosphatase 2A) [8] (Figure 1). Finally, experiments on cultured cancer cells reveal that Hippo signalling pathway components are required for E-cadherin-dependent contact inhibition of proliferation, and that expression of E-cadherin in breast cancer cells restores the density-dependent regulation of YAP nuclear exclusion [23]. In summary both TJ and AJ protein complexes, depending on the cellular context and experimental approach, have been shown to play a crucial role in controlling the subcellular localization and activity of YAP, through both Hippo pathway-dependent and -independent mechanisms.

RhoA-dependent control of gene expression: interplay with junctional proteins?

The notion that actin dynamics affects the activity of transcription factors, and hence gene expression, was first raised by experiments showing that the polymerization state of actin controls the activity of SRF (serum response factor) [24]. Actin polymerization and dynamics is regulated at multiple levels, and a major role is played by Rho family GTPases: RhoA, Rac1 and Cdc42 (cell division cycle 42). Indeed, SRF activity and subcellular localization was eventually shown to depend on RhoA activity. Intriguingly, Rho GTPases are regulated by several junctional proteins, including p120-ctn, E-cadherin, afadin, ZO-3, cingulin, paracingulin, AMOT and PAR-6, through different mechanisms, including binding to activators [GEFs (guanine-nucleotide-exchange factors)] and inhibitors [GAPs (GTPase-activating proteins)], and post-translational modifications [25]. This raises the possibility that the junction-dependent regulation of Rho family GTPases may be an additional mechanism through which junctional proteins control gene expression and cell proliferation.

This hypothesis has been validated by studies on cingulin, a cytoplasmic TJ protein that recruits and inactivates the RhoA activator GEF-H1 at TJs, thus resulting in a down-regulation of RhoA activity in confluent monolayers [26] (Figure 2). In different types of cultured cell models, knockout or depletion of cingulin affects gene expression, for example the expression of claudin-2, and cell proliferation [27,28]. The proliferation phenotype and the up-regulation of claudin-2 expression in cingulin-depleted kidney cells are rescued by inhibition of RhoA, indicating that some of the effects of cingulin depletion on gene expression are due to its GEF-H1-dependent regulation of RhoA activity [28] (Figure 2). Interestingly, ZONAB activity is also regulated by GEF-H1, indicating that GEF-H1 and ZONAB form a signalling module that mediates Rho-regulated cyclin D1 promoter activation and expression [29] (Figure 2).

It should be noted that the relationship between junctions and Rho family GTPases is dual. Not only do AJC proteins control Rho GTPases, but the AJC is itself a major target of Rho family GTPases, which are crucially required for its formation and maintenance, through remodelling of the actin cytoskeleton, and activation of the PAR-3–PAR-6–aPKC (atypical protein kinase C) polarity complex. Furthermore, extrinsic cues act on junctions through Rho GTPases. For example, TGFβ (transforming growth factor β)-dependent EMT (epithelial–mesenchymal transition) leads to the disruption of junctions through the PAR-6-dependent ubiquitination and degradation of RhoA [30].

Finally, another example illustrating the multiple routes through which Rho GTPases control cell physiology was the recent demonstration that RhoA/ROCK (Rho-associated kinase)-dependent cytoskeletal tension and stress fibre formation control the nucleo-cytoplasmic shuttling of the transcription factor YAP, independently of the Hippo pathway [31]. Since YAP and TAZ also interact with and are regulated by junctional and polarity proteins (see above), these observations suggest the existence of a complex intriguing interplay between junctions, the actin cytoskeleton and transcriptional regulation.

Conclusions

The cytoplasmic domain of TJs and AJs is a hot spot for signalling, since it provides a platform to recruit transcription factors and other essential signalling molecules, such as regulators of GTPases. Moreover, several junctional proteins can shuttle to the nucleus, and bind to and tune the activity of transcription factors. The signalling functions of some junctional proteins have been validated by studies on animal-knockout models and diseases, demonstrating that the AJC is essential to control gene expression and cell proliferation in epithelial cells at the organism level.

How do junctions regulate gene expression and cell proliferation? A likely scenario, on the basis of the information currently available, is that when differentiated epithelial cells form stable junctions within confluent monolayers, cell proliferation is down-regulated through the sequestration of signalling molecules at junctions. Conversely, disruption of junctions following intrinsic or extrinsic stimuli, for example the activation of the Wnt pathway, leads to a redistribution of junctional proteins, and transcriptional activation of proliferation-related genes. Phosphorylation appears to be a general mechanism that promotes the cytoplasmic retention of junction-associated signalling proteins. Since the configuration and regulation of signalling pathways may depend on cell type and differentiated/pathological cell properties, such a scenario may not be always applicable, underlining the importance of hypothesis validation in different cell culture and animal models, whenever possible. Moreover, how the organization of the actin cytoskeleton controls the localization of transcription factors remains an interesting question to be investigated.

In summary, the AJC responds to a variety of extracellular and intracellular signalling cues through many of its protein components, and functions to integrate these signals into co-ordinated changes in cell shape, adhesion and proliferation.

Summary

- *The AJC (TJs and AJs) has canonical roles in cell adhesion and barrier function of epithelia, but also plays a major role in signalling.*
- *Several TJ and AJ proteins can shuttle between the cytoplasm and the nucleus, depending on cell density, culture conditions and different extrinsic or intrinsic stimuli.*
- *TJ and AJ proteins can bind to and sequester transcription factors and signalling proteins at cell–cell junctions.*
- *The subcellular localization of the transcription factors ZONAB, YAP and other nuclear proteins correlates with cell density, and is regulated by junctional and cytoskeletal proteins.*
- *Transcription factors that shuttle between the AJC and the nucleus, such as ZONAB and YAP, are critical modulators of cell proliferation, cell differentiation and growth.*
- *The small GTPase RhoA regulates cell proliferation and gene expression by controlling the activity and nuclear localization of the transcription factors SRF, ZONAB and YAP.*
- *The ability of AJC proteins, such as cingulin, to control the activity of Rho family GTPases is one of the mechanisms through which the AJC regulates gene expression and cell proliferation.*

We thank the Swiss National Foundation, the State of Geneva and the Section of Biology of the Faculty of Sciences of the University of Geneva for support, and Serge Paschoud for comments on the chapter. We apologize for not citing a large number of relevant publications, due to a limitation in the number of references.

References

1. Meng, W. and Takeichi, M. (2009) Adherens junction: molecular architecture and regulation. Cold Spring Harbor Perspect. Biol., doi:10.1101/cshperspect.a002899
2. Anderson, J.M., Van Itallie, C.M. and Fanning, A.S. (2004) Setting up a selective barrier at the apical junction complex. Curr. Opin. Cell Biol. **16**, 140–145
3. Shin, K., Fogg, V.C. and Margolis, B. (2006) Tight junctions and cell polarity. Annu. Rev. Cell Dev. Biol. **22**, 207–235
4. McCrea, P.D., Gu, D. and Balda, M.S. (2009) Junctional music that the nucleus hears: cell–cell contact signalling and the modulation of gene activity. Cold Spring Harb Perspect. Biol. **1**, a002923
5. Behrens, J., von Kries, J.P., Kuhl, M., Bruhn, L., Wedlich, D., Grosschedl, R. and Birchmeier, W. (1996) Functional interaction of beta-catenin with the transcription factor LEF-1. Nature **382**, 638–642
6. Kelly, K.F., Spring, C.M., Otchere, A.A. and Daniel, J.M. (2004) NLS-dependent nuclear localization of p120ctn is necessary to relieve Kaiso-mediated transcriptional repression. J Cell Sci. **117**, 2675–2686
7. Vasioukhin, V., Bauer, C., Degenstein, L., Wise, B. and Fuchs, E. (2001) Hyperproliferation and defects in epithelial polarity upon conditional ablation of α-catenin in skin. Cell **104**, 605–617

8. Schlegelmilch, K., Mohseni, M., Kirak, O., Pruszak, J., Rodriguez, J.R., Zhou, D., Kreger, B.T., Vasioukhin, V., Avruch, J., Brummelkamp, T.R. and Camargo, F.D. (2011) Yap1 acts downstream of α-catenin to control epidermal proliferation. Cell **144**, 782–795

9. Silvis, M.R., Kreger, B.T., Lien, W.H., Klezovitch, O., Rudakova, G.M., Camargo, F.D., Lantz, D.M., Seykora, J.T., and Vasioukhin, V. (2011) α-Catenin is a tumor suppressor that controls cell accumulation by regulating the localization and activity of the transcriptional coactivator Yap1. Sci. Signalling **4**, ra33

10. Balda, M.S. and Matter, K. (2000) The tight junction protein ZO-1 and an interacting transcription factor regulate ErbB-2 expression. EMBO J **19**, 2024–2033

11. Sourisseau, T., Georgiadis, A., Tsapara, A., Ali, R.R., Pestell, R., Matter, K. and Balda, M.S. (2006) Regulation of PCNA and cyclin D1 expression and epithelial morphogenesis by the ZO-1-regulated transcription factor ZONAB/DbpA. Mol. Cell Biol. **26**, 2387–2398

12. Kavanagh, E., Buchert, M., Tsapara, A., Choquet, A., Balda, M.S., Hollande, F. and Matter, K. (2006) Functional interaction between the ZO-1-interacting transcription factor ZONAB/DbpA and the RNA processing factor symplekin. J. Cell Sci. **119**, 5098–5105

13. Xing, H., Mayhew, C.N., Cullen, K.E., Park-Sarge, O.K. and Sarge, K.D. (2004) HSF1 modulation of Hsp70 mRNA polyadenylation via interaction with symplekin. J. Biol. Chem. **279**, 10551–10555

14. Buchert, M., Darido, C., Lagerqvist, E., Sedello, A., Cazevieille, C., Buchholz, F., Bourgaux, J.F., Pannequin, J., Joubert, D. and Hollande, F. (2009) The symplekin/ZONAB complex inhibits intestinal cell differentiation by the repression of AML1/Runx1. Gastroenterology **137**, 156–164

15. Huerta, M., Munoz, R., Tapia, R., Soto-Reyes, E., Ramirez, L., Recillas-Targa, F., Gonzalez-Mariscal, L. and Lopez-Bayghen, E. (2007) Cyclin D1 is transcriptionally down-regulated by ZO-2 via an E box and the transcription factor c-Myc. Mol. Biol. Cell **18**, 4826–4836

16. Traweger, A., Fuchs, R., Krizbai, I.A., Weiger, T.M., Bauer, H.C. and Bauer, H. (2003) The tight junction protein ZO-2 localizes to the nucleus and interacts with the heterogeneous nuclear ribonucleoprotein scaffold attachment factor-B. J. Biol. Chem. **278**, 2692–2700

17. Betanzos, A., Huerta, M., Lopez-Bayghen, E., Azuara, E., Amerena, J. and Gonzalez-Mariscal, L. (2004) The tight junction protein ZO-2 associates with Jun, Fos and C/EBP transcription factors in epithelial cells. Exp. Cell Res. **292**, 51–66

18. Capaldo, C.T., Koch, S., Kwon, M., Laur, O., Parkos, C.A. and Nusrat, A. (2011) Tight function zonula occludens-3 regulates cyclin D1-dependent cell proliferation. Mol. Biol. Cell **22**, 1677–1685

19. Zhao, B., Li, L., Lu, Q., Wang, L.H., Liu, C.Y., Lei, Q. and Guan, K.L. (2011) Angiomotin is a novel Hippo pathway component that inhibits YAP oncoprotein. Genes Dev. **25**, 51–63

20. Wang, W., Huang, J. and Chen, J. (2011) Angiomotin-like proteins associate with and negatively regulate YAP1. J. Biol. Chem. **286**, 4364–4370

21. Cordenonsi, M., Zanconato, F., Azzolin, L., Forcato, M., Rosato, A., Frasson, C., Inui, M., Montagner, M., Parenti, A.R., Poletti, A. et al. (2011) The Hippo transducer TAZ confers cancer stem cell-related traits on breast cancer cells. Cell **147**, 759–772

22. Oka, T., Remue, E., Meerschaert, K., Vanloo, B., Boucherie, C., Gfeller, D., Bader, G.D., Sidhu, S.S., Vandekerckhove, J., Gettemans, J. and Sudol, M. (2010) Functional complexes between YAP2 and ZO-2 are PDZ domain-dependent, and regulate YAP2 nuclear localization and signalling. Biochem. J. **432**, 461–472

23. Kim, N.G., Koh, E., Chen, X. and Gumbiner, B.M. (2011) E-cadherin mediates contact inhibition of proliferation through Hippo signalling-pathway components. Proc. Natl. Acad. Sci. U.S.A. **108**, 11930–11935

24. Sotiropoulos, A., Gineitis, D., Copeland, J. and Treisman, R. (1999) Signal-regulated activation of serum response factor is mediated by changes in actin dynamics. Cell **98**, 159–169

25. Citi, S., Spadaro, D., Schneider, Y., Stutz, J. and Pulimeno, P. (2011) Regulation of small GTPases at epithelial cell-cell junctions. Mol. Membr. Biol. **28**, 427–444

26. Aijaz, S., D'Atri, F., Citi, S., Balda, M.S. and Matter, K. (2005) Binding of GEF-H1 to the tight junction-associated adaptor cingulin results in inhibition of Rho signalling and G1/S phase transition. Dev. Cell **8**, 777–786

27. Guillemot, L., Hammar, E., Kaister, C., Ritz, J., Caille, D., Jond, L., Bauer, C., Meda, P. and Citi, S. (2004) Disruption of the cingulin gene does not prevent tight junction formation but alters gene expression. J. Cell Sci. **117**, 5245–5256

28. Guillemot, L. and Citi, S. (2006) Cingulin regulates claudin-2 expression and cell proliferation through the small GTPase RhoA. Mol. Biol. Cell **17**, 3569–3577

29. Nie, M., Aijaz, S., Leefa Chong San, I.V., Balda, M.S. and Matter, K. (2009) The Y-box factor ZONAB/DbpA associates with GEF-H1/Lfc and mediates Rho-stimulated transcription. EMBO Rep. **10**, 1125–1131

30. Ozdamar, B., Bose, R., Barrios-Rodiles, M., Wang, H.R., Zhang, Y. and Wrana, J.L. (2005) Regulation of the polarity protein Par6 by TGFβ receptors controls epithelial cell plasticity. Science **307**, 1603–1609

31. Dupont, S., Morsut, L., Aragona, M., Enzo, E., Giulitti, S., Cordenonsi, M., Zanconato, F., Le Digabel, J., Forcato, M., Bicciato, S. et al. (2011) Role of YAP/TAZ in mechanotransduction. Nature **474**, 179–183

© The Authors Journal compilation © 2012 Biochemical Society
Essays Biochem. (2012) **53**, 95–109: doi: 10.1042/BSE0530095

8

Apicobasal polarity and cell proliferation during development

Nitin Sabherwal and Nancy Papalopulu

Faculty of Life Sciences, Michael Smith Building, University of Manchester, Oxford Road, Manchester M13 9PT, U.K.

Abstract

Cell polarization and cell division are two fundamental cellular processes. The mechanisms that establish and maintain cell polarity and the mechanisms by which cells progress through the cell cycle are now fairly well understood following decades of experimental work. There is also increasing evidence that the polarization state of a cell affects its proliferative properties. The challenge now is to understand how these two phenomena are mechanistically connected. The aim of the present chapter is to provide an overview of the evidence of cross-talk between apicobasal polarity and proliferation, and the current state of knowledge of the precise mechanism by which this cross-talk is achieved.

Introduction: apicobasal polarity and cell proliferation

Polarization can be defined as the asymmetrical distribution of cellular components. Most, if not all, cells are polarized in one way or another. Cells polarize in order to reduce intracellular disorder and vectorize cellular activities, such as membrane trafficking and cellular secretion. In the context of epithelial tissues,

*Correspondence may be addressed to either author (email Nitin.Sabherwal@
manchester.ac.uk or Nancy.Papalopulu@manchester.ac.uk).*

polarization of cells perpendicular to the plane of tissue results in apicobasal polarity.

Apicobasally polarized epithelial cells show polarity not only in their plasma membrane, but also within their cortex, the cytoskeleton-rich cytoplasm lying underneath the membrane. Cortical polarity results from the polarization of actin cytoskeleton and its associated proteins. Unlike in non-polar cells where plasma membrane constituents are in motion and intermixing continuously, membrane polarization results in the generation of distinct apical and basolateral plasma membrane domains. These domains do not mix, due to the presence of AJCs (apical junctional complexes; composed of adherens junctions, and tight or septate junctions), resulting in differences with respect to their protein and lipid content. Therefore the formation of AJCs is thought to be essential for establishing and maintaining polarity, although, in some instances, cells have been reported to establish and maintain polarity in isolation, in the absence of cell–cell contacts [1].

Apicobasal polarity is established and maintained by the antagonistic interactions between apical and basolateral protein complexes, primarily mediated through the phosphorylation reactions of the kinases involved in polarity [2]. The key apical complex is the aPKC (atypical protein kinase C)–PAR (PARtioning defective) complex, consisting of an atypical serine/threonine protein kinase (aPKC), along with two PDZ [PSD-95 (postsynaptic density 95), Dlg (discs large) and ZO-1]-domain-containing scaffold proteins (PAR-3 and PAR-6). These three proteins form a functional unit, which is essential for the establishment and maintenance of the apical domain. The apical Crumbs complex, consisting of the transmembrane protein Crumbs and its associated cytoplasmic proteins PALS1 (protein associated with lin seven 1) and PATJ (PALS1-associated tight junction protein), is also required for apical membrane establishment. Basolateral kinases PAR-1 and PAR-4 are necessary for basolateral membrane identity. Like PAR-1 and PAR-4, the basolateral Scribble complex [containing Scribble, Lgl (lethal giant larvae) and Dlg (discs large)] is involved in the maintenance of apicobasal polarity by negatively regulating the expansion of the apical membrane. These molecular complexes are highly conserved between various systems and contexts [3].

Like cell polarity, cell proliferation is a fundamental and equally important cellular process. Cell division leads to cell proliferation and tissue growth, and is controlled by the cell cycle. The cell cycle can be defined as a process whereby a cell divides [in M (mitotic)-phase] after its genome has duplicated [in S (synthetic)-phase]. These two phases are alternated with the presence of two gap phases (G_1 after M-phase and G_2 after S-phase), which function as the preparatory phases for the upcoming events in M- and S-phases. The key regulators of the cell cycle are the CDKs (cyclin-dependent kinases), which are positively regulated by cyclins and negatively regulated by CDKIs (CDK inhibitors). Various combinations of CDKs, cyclins and CDKIs constitute the molecular check-points, which serve as the regulatory points for the cells to leave one phase of the cell cycle and enter the next. While the basic machinery of the cell cycle is fairly well understood and can be viewed as an autonomous entity, it is clear that it receives inputs from the cellular environment both during development and in disease, in the form of extracellular signalling. The G_1-phase is the key phase where extracellular signals impinge on the cell-cycle machinery, to instruct the cell to proceed through division or not [4]. In addition, as we will discuss in detail below, the structure of the cell, for example, whether it is polarized or not can affect its division properties.

During development and tissue homoeostasis, the cell cycle needs to be controlled in order to prevent premature or complete depletion of progenitor cells, or conversely, uncontrolled growth. There are two main ways in which the cell cycle may be affected: cells may exit the cell cycle prematurely or remain in the cell cycle longer than the normal schedule. Alternatively, the kinetics of the cell cycle, such as the speed or proportional length of G_1, can also be altered. Both of these can have profound effects on cell numbers and the differentiation state of a tissue. Interestingly, these are not mutually exclusive possibilities, as emerging evidence indicates that altered cell-cycle kinetics may affect cell-cycle exit [5].

Model systems for studying polarity in conjunction with cell proliferation

Model systems, from yeast to higher vertebrates, have been invaluable for elucidating the mechanisms of polarity and cell proliferation control. Although each of these processes can be studied separately, in the present chapter we will limit our discussion to the model systems that have been used for elucidating the mechanisms that control polarity and cell proliferation in relation to each other, as these would offer the most promise for understanding the molecular intersection of these two biological processes. These include *Drosophila* NBs (neuroblasts) and imaginal discs as the invertebrate model systems, and mouse and *Xenopus* neuroectoderm as the vertebrate models. Work on *Caenorhabditis elegans*, a model system which has been instrumental in the initial identification of genes involved in polarity, its establishment and maintenance and its role in spindle orientation, will be discussed elsewhere in the volume (see Chapter 1).

Drosophila NBs and imaginal discs

Drosophila NBs are stem cells for the development of the central nervous system and one of the key invertebrate model systems for studying cell polarity, asymmetric cell division and stem cell self-renewal. NBs divide asymmetrically to generate two cells of unequal developmental potential: an apicobasally polarized cell, which is identical with the mother stem cell, and stays in the cell cycle, and a non-polarized cell, called the GMC (ganglion mother cell), which divides only once more to terminally differentiate into two neurons or glial cells [6]. NBs show all the hallmarks of cortical apicobasal polarity, in the form of apical localization of a PAR complex and basolateral localization of the Lgl–Dlg–Scribble complex. A number of critical RNAs and proteins are associated with

this basolateral complex, such as Numb, Prospero and Brat. These are collectively called fate determinants (Figure 1). Both apical and basolateral polarity
protein complexes are necessary for their localization to the basal side of the
neuroblast. Before cell division, alignment of spindle parallel to the apicobasal
axis ensures the correct segregation of these fate determinants in the GMC [6].
The key function of the fate determinants is to inhibit cell division and promote
differentiation of GMCs. Numb acts as a Notch inhibitor, therefore the unequal
inheritance of Numb generates Notch asymmetry between the daughter NB
and the GMC. The GMC has low Notch activity and shows low proliferation
potential [7]. Prospero, upon asymmetric division, is relieved from its adaptor

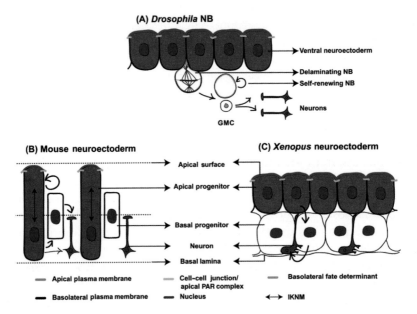

Figure 1. Key model systems of polarity and proliferation
(**A**) *Drosophila* NBs (neuroblasts) are a model of polarized neural stem cells. A NB delaminates
from the ventral neuroectoderm but still maintains its apicobasal polarity. It divides asymetrically
to self-renew and give rise to a non-polar GMC (ganglion mother cell), which further divides terminally to differentiate into two neurons. (**B**) The VZ (ventricular zone) of the mouse embryonic
cortex/mouse neuroectoderm contains polarized APs (apical progenitors) which divide both
symetrically to self-renew and asymmetrically to produce either a BP (basal progenitor) or a neuron, along with another AP. BPs mainly divide terminally to differentiate into neurons. Other layers of mouse cortex [SVZ (subventricular zone), IZ (intermediate zone) and CP (cortical plate)]
have not been shown in the scheme for the sake of simplicity. (**C**) *Xenopus* neuroectoderm presents with a unique system. This ectoderm is bilayered with outer layer cells being apicobasally
polar and inner cells non-polar. Inner cells are generated by asymmetric divisions of outer polar
cells, which stay as long-term neural progenitors. Only the inner non-polar cells have the capacity to differentiate into primary neurons. Free arrows in the schemes indicate what possible fates
the cells can adopt on their division. Another invertebrate model system of polarity and proliferation is the *Drosophila* imaginal discs, which are sacs of epithelial cells and show all the hallmarks
of apicobasal polarity. Schematically they are similar to the *Drosophila* ventral neuroectoderm and
are not shown here. In all of the systems described, polar cells have a different proliferation
potential than non-polar cells, and manipulating their polarity alters their proliferation properties.

protein Miranda, enters the GMC nucleus and acts as a transcription factor [8,9]. Nuclear translocation of Prospero acts as a binary switch between a proliferating NB and a differentiating GMC. It represses genes required for stem cell renewal and cell cycle, such as String/Cdc25 (Cdc is cell division cycle), cyclin A, cyclin E and E2F factor, and activates differentiation genes such as even skipped and fushi tarazu [10]. Brat functions similarly, but at a post-transcriptional level; it inhibits the translation of Myc protein, a key regulator of cell-cycle growth [11].

Drosophila imaginal discs are another well-characterized experimental system to study cell proliferation and polarity. Several mutational screens for proliferation mutants have been performed using imaginal discs. These are larval epithelial sacs that contribute to adult cuticular structures. Imaginal disc precursors are small groups of embryonic ectodermal cells that are set aside during embryogenesis as clusters of approximately 20–50 cells. They proliferate extensively to their final sizes of 20000–50000 cells and invaginate to form the imaginal discs during larval development. Towards the end of the larval stage imaginal disc cells are committed to specific fates. During metamorphosis, while larval cells enter apoptosis, the imaginal discs undergo major morphogenetic changes to form the adult legs, wings, eyes, antennae, head capsule, halteres and genital organs. Because of their epithelial architecture, proliferation potential and well-described development, imaginal discs (in particular wing and eye discs) serve as important model systems for studying proliferation control of apicobasally polarized epithelial cells. As these cells proliferate during the larval stages, the issues pertaining to maternal contribution are avoided. They are also highly amenable to mosaic analysis as well as measurements of doubling times because of the ease of inducing clones via mitotic recombination [12].

Vertebrate embryonic neuroepithilium/mouse and *Xenopus* embryonic neuroectoderm

The mouse embryonic cortex is the most widely studied vertebrate model to understand the effect of polarity on the balance of proliferation versus differentiation. It contains several cellular layers, namely VZ (ventricular zone), SVZ (subventricular zone), IZ (intermediate zone) and the CP (cortical plate), which are identified on the basis of their locations, the cell types they contain and the markers they express. The VZ layer faces the cortical lumen, whereas SVZ, IZ and CP layers lie underneath the VZ. The VZ is composed of apicobasally polarized progenitors (apical progenitors), showing apical aPKC with tight and adherens junctions at the most apical end of the lateral plasma membrane and integrin receptors in the basal plasma membrane. They also show a pseudostratified epithelial architecture, undergo IKNM (interkinetic nuclear migration) and their nuclei divide on the apical side of cells (Figure 1). Before the onset of neurogenesis, apical progenitors divide symmetrically to generate more apical progenitors and expand their population. With the progression of neurogenesis, they increasingly switch to asymmetric neurogenic division, giving rise to a polar apical progenitor and a non-polar neuronal cell, as well as asymmetric proliferative divisions, replenishing themselves and also giving rise to basally located non-polar BPs (basal progenitors) (Figure 1). BPs, located in both the VZ and SVZ, divide symmetrically to differentiate into neurons; they rarely self-renew. Neurons generated from apical progenitors and BPs migrate away from the VZ and SVZ to the underlying neuronal layers (IZ and CP) [13]. With the development of cortex, BPs are gradually depleted, whereas the apical progenitors are the only progenitors with unlimited self-renewing capacity [14].

With the progression of neurogenesis from E11–E17 (E is embryonic day), the cell-cycle length of neural progenitors increases significantly, accompanied by a lengthening of the G_1-phase [15]. Both apical progenitors and BPs also differ with respect to the G_1-phase length [16]. Both gain- and loss-of-function experiments with regulators of the G_1 length (cyclin D/CDK4 and cyclin E/CDK2) have shown that G_1 lengthening is a cause, rather than a consequence, of neurogenesis [17,18]. It is primarily linked with the generation of BPs by apical progenitors and also associated with a switch from proliferative to neurogenic divisions [17–19]. Shortening of the G_1-phase by overexpression of G_1 kinase complexes increases symmetrical expansions of both apical progenitors and BPs at the expense of neurogenic divisions. Inversely, increasing G_1 length by RNAi (RNA interference) knockdown of the same complexes was shown to promote neurogenesis at the expense of proliferative progenitor divisions [17,18]. These experiments led to the formulation of the 'cell-cycle length hypothesis' [19] which postulates that the length of the G_1-phase is the determining factor for a cell to stay as a proliferative progenitor, or to undergo differentiation. The hypothesis is that a longer G_1 gives enough time to the differentiation determinants to accumulate and mature, acting on the newly post-mitotic cells to push them towards differentiation. Thus apical progenitors and BPs in the mouse cortex differ not only in their polarity status, but also in their proliferation and cell-cycle properties, making this an excellent model system to study the links between polarity and proliferation.

The neuroectoderm of the *Xenopus* embryo during gastrulation and early phases of neurulation, provides another vertebrate model of polarity and proliferation. Before neural tube closure, the ectoderm is bilayered, consisting of a superficial cell layer of apicobasally polarized cells, overlaying a deep layer of cells, which are non-polar (Figure 1). The polarized cells exhibit all the hallmarks of embryonic epithelial polarity, such as the apical localization of aPKC and basolateral localization of Lgl and PAR-1. The polarity of superficial cells is established and maintained by the classical regulators of polarity, aPKC and Lgl [20]. Cells in these two layers are intrinsically different with respect to their cell fates: while the deep cells are able to differentiate into primary neurons, superficial cells stay as long-term progenitors [21]. Superficial cells can be compared with the apical progenitors in mouse cortex (but show no pseudostratified architecture and no apparent IKNM), whereas the deep cells are akin to the basal progenitors. This simple bilayered architecture of *Xenopus* neuroectoderm makes it an excellent model system to study the effects of polarity on proliferation.

Evidence that polarity and proliferation are linked

Various observations indicate that polarity and proliferation are linked in normal development and disease. From the evidence presented above, it is clear that during the development of the *Drosophila* and vertebrate nervous system, non-polarized progenitors are closer to cell-cycle exit than polarized progenitors. In the mouse cortex, polarized and non-polarized progenitors also differ in their cell-cycle kinetics, such as the length of G_1 [16].

In disease, it is notable that approximately 90% of the human cancers originate from the apicobasally polarized epithelial cells. Indeed, aberrant proliferation and concomitant loss of apicobasal polarity are the most salient feature of human cancers [22].

Molecular data support these phenomenological observations. A genetic screen in *Drosophila* to uncover novel tumour suppressor genes identified genes, which were later found to be integral components of the apicobasal polarity machinery, such as Lgl [23,24]. Components of apicobasal polarity are also known to function as proto-oncogenes or tumour suppressors. Loss- or gain-of-function mutations in these genes are associated with uncontrolled proliferation during cancer progression and stem cell renewal [22,25]. Last, but not the least, polarity molecules also regulate the Hippo pathway, a key sensor of cellular growth and division, to control cell proliferation [26].

Mechanisms linking polarity and proliferation in *Drosophila* models

Drosophila has been a key developmental model system to study the mechanistic links between polarity and proliferation. During *Drosophila* neural development, non-polarized GMCs formed after the asymmetric divisions of polarized NBs receive the full complement of basal fate determinants (Numb, Prospero and Brat). GMCs generated from the loss-of-function NB mutants for cell-fate determinants cannot exit the cell cycle, show NB-like properties and keep proliferating, giving rise to ectopic NBs and brain tumours in flies [10,11,27]. These results put the emphasis on proteins of the basolateral complex for cell-cycle exit regulation, as GMCs lack the apically localized aPKC–PAR complex.

The situation is more complex in the polarized self-renewing progenitor, the NB, which contains the full complement of both apical and basolateral polarity proteins. What keeps them in a proliferative/self-renewal and non-differentiation state despite having the basal fate determinants? The answer lies in the differential subcellular localization of fate determinants; for example, Prospero is nuclear and thus active as a transcription factor only in GMCs (Figure 1) [9]. What then regulates the differential localization and activity of fate determinants in NBs versus GMCs? The key molecule regulating this process is the apical polarity kinase aPKC, the first protein identified to regulate self-renewal of NBs [28]. The role of aPKC in NB self-renewal involves aPKC phosphorylating and inactivating fate determinants, such as Lgl, Numb and Miranda [29–31]. aPKC also regulates the orientation of the mitotic spindle. Thus an indirect control of aPKC over fate determinants could also be exerted by controlling the distribution of the basolateral complex by virtue of orienting the mitotic spindle [32]. These data suggest that aPKC has an indirect role in preventing NB differentiation by negatively regulating the activity of basolateral fate determinants. But does aPKC have a more direct role in NB proliferation?

Some evidence suggests that the role of aPKC in NB proliferation might result from aPKC actively speeding up the cell cycle. NB mutants with zygotic loss of aPKC show reduced cellular proliferation [28,33]. A similar phenotype was observed for the loss-of-function mutant of Dap160 (dynamin-associated protein 160), a positive regulator of aPKC. Reduced proliferation in Dap160 mutants was attributed to a prolonged cell cycle due to longer interphase [34]. Conversely, NB-specific overexpression of membrane-targeted aPKC or loss-of-function of negative regulators of aPKC [such as the phosphatase Twins/ PP2A (protein phosphatase 2A)] induced ectopic NB self-renewal and supernumerary NBs [33,35]. Similar to the gain of apically localized aPKC, loss of basolateral Lgl results in hyperproliferation of NBs [33]. Very importantly, Lgl mutant NBs show ectopic cortical localization of aPKC, and the hyperproliferation phenotype of these mutants can be fully rescued in an Lgl/aPKC double mutant. These data suggest that the role of aPKC in NB proliferation is not only direct, but may be dominant as well, and it is sufficient to turn GMCs into NBs. However, biochemical evidence is needed to understand how aPKC may exert a direct role on proliferation and this will be elaborated further below.

This 'dominant role of apical aPKC in NB renewal' hypothesis has recently been vigorously tested. In Mud (Mushroom body defective) NB mutants, apical localization of PAR-3 and aPKC is normal, but spindle alignment parallel with apicobasal polarity is disrupted, leading to ectopic symmetric divisions and proliferation of mutant NBs. Prospero overexpression in Mud mutant NBs results in striking depletion of ectopic NBs. If the role of aPKC was dominant in determining NB cell fate, overexpressing Prospero should have no effect in rescuing the phenotype. This observation led to the idea that it is the ratio of apical/basal polarity markers that determines the NB/GMC identity; while a higher apical/ basal ratio promotes NB identity, a higher basal/apical ratio promotes GMC identity [36].

In imaginal discs, similar to NBs, loss of aPKC leads to the loss of polarity and proliferation in the eye disc cells [28,32]. Conversely, loss of basolateral proteins Lgl/Dlg/Scribble, is associated with overproliferation and loss of tissue architecture in the wing imaginal disc cells [24]. Ectopic growth in the imaginal disc tissues by gain of apical aPKC or loss of basolateral Lgl/Dlg/Scribble is more actively associated with positive changes in cell-cycle progression.

Overproliferation in *Drosophila* mutants for Lgl/Dlg/Scribble in the developing eyes, results from the ectopic S-phase entry of the nuclei, which is accounted for by the negative regulation of cyclin E, the key regulator of G_1-to-S-phase entry during cell cycle, by Lgl/Dlg/Scribble [37]. This is consistent with the role of the Lgl/Dlg/Scribble polarity protein complex in cancer, which is discussed in Chapter 11.

Imaginal disc cells have also paved the way for elucidating the control of cell proliferation by polarity molecules via regulation of the hyperplastic tumour suppressor Hippo pathway. This is a kinase cascade pathway, which negatively regulates the activity of a downstream oncogenic transcriptional co-activator Yki (Yorkie), by direct phosphorylation and cytoplasmic sequestration [26]. Although primarily cytoplasmic, an active apical pool of Hippo kinase complex has been reported [38,39], which is positively regulated by the upstream apical scaffold protein complex MEK, consisting of Merlin (M), Expanded (E) and Kibra (K) [26,40]. The Hippo pathway is reviewed in Chapter 9; therefore it will be only briefly touched upon in the present chapter in the context of polarity. Overexpression of aPKC or loss of Lgl in the eye epithelial tissue causes cytoplasmic mislocalization of apical Hippo and its co-localization with its negative regulator RASSF (Ras-associated factor), dampening Hippo signalling and enhancing proliferation [38]. How does Lgl/aPKC deregulate the Hippo pathway? Human Kibra is an aPKC direct phosphorylation target [41]. Kibra phosphorylation and deregulation by aPKC could be a possiblility, leading to apical loss of Hippo complex. Apical Crumbs also regulates cellular proliferation via regulating the levels and apical localization of Expanded protein. Crumbs directly binds to Expanded and this binding also leads to the phosphorylation of Expanded [42,43], although the kinase involved is not known. It is possible that aPKC is the kinase, phosphorylating apical Expanded.

Interestingly, there are examples of mechanistically separable effects of polarity components on polarity and proliferation. In *Drosophila* eye imaginal discs, Lgl mutant cells in the wild-type surroundings show ectopic proliferation via up-regulated Hippo pathway. Clonal analysis of these mutant cells had shown that they exhibited no effect on polarity, which was attributed to the presence of maternal Lgl protein. However, the same cells, when grown until pupal stage, showed loss of polarity. Together these observations led to the idea that Lgl affected proliferation and polarity at different thresholds; higher levels of Lgl are needed for inhibiting proliferation, whereas lower levels are required for its function in polarity maintenance [38,44]. Separable effects on polarity and proliferation of Crumbs were also shown by the gain-of-function mutants of Crumbs[icd] (intracellular domain of Crumbs). Separate subdomains within the intracellular domain of Crumbs were shown to be responsible for its function in proliferation via the Hippo pathway, and in polarity through its interaction with the PAR–aPKC complex [45]. Further examples of such functional separation are provided by LKB1/PAR-4 and Dlg [46,47]. These examples add an additional layer of complexity in deciphering the direct effects of polarity components in proliferation.

Mechanisms linking polarity and proliferation in the vertebrate neuroepithelium

As cortical development proceeds in mouse (from E11 to E17), neural progenitors perform more neurogenic than proliferative divisions [13]. During this period, apical polarity markers such as PAR-3, PAR-6 and aPKC show significant reduction in their staining intensity, indicating that proliferation and the amount of apical polarity markers are correlatively linked. Loss-of-function of endogenous PAR-3 and PAR-6 blocks cortical progenitor expansion and overexpression of PAR-6 results in clonal expansion of apical progenitors, both *in vitro* and *in vivo*, without having any obvious effect on the expansion of BPs. This expansion is achieved by means of an increase in the number of symmetric proliferative divisions, without affecting their overall cell-cycle length [48].

Nevertheless, since it is also known that polarized and non-polar progenitors in mouse neuroepithelium have different cell-cycle lengths [16], one possibility is that, in some instances, polarity affects cell fate via changes in the cell-cycle length, which is known to be associated with cell-fate changes [19]. However, mechanistic evidence for this is currently lacking. Some answers in this direction might come from the experiments in *Xenopus* ectoderm. Here, inhibiting aPKC leads to enhanced differentiation, whereas the overexpression of membrane-tethered aPKC (aPKC-CAAX) leads to the inhibition of differentiation and enhanced proliferation of the entire ectoderm. This suggested that aPKC is a key regulator of proliferation [49], consistent with results in other organisms. Further experiments in *Xenopus* showed that the effects of aPKC-CAAX on differentiation and proliferation were phenocopied by a nuclear kinase construct of aPKC [49]. This suggested that aPKC itself might shuttle between the membrane and the nucleus to implement its effect on cell fate, possibly via direct phosphorylation of nuclear proteins. Follow-up experiments showed that aPKC overexpression leads to faster cell cycle of the progenitors, without affecting their growth fraction (N. Sabherwal and N. Papalopulu, unpublished work). So in *Xenopus* neuroepithelium, the effects of aPKC on proliferation may be mediated via cell-cycle changes. Such changes by aPKC overexpression might lead to alterations in the proliferative compared with differentiative divisions of both apical progenitors and BPs, as has been observed for mouse cortical progenitors. The mechanistic details of these changes are still under investigation and will be revealed in future publications. Finally in this system, polarity molecules, such as PAR-1, can also control the orientation of division, and their manipulation can also affect the fate of the cells [50].

Conclusions and unanswered questions

Model systems described above have provided a wealth of information on how the polarization state of a cell regulates its proliferation. It regulates the mode of division of cells (symmetric compared with asymmetric) and thereby affects their cell-cycle exit properties. It may regulate their cell-cycle kinetics, which has also been shown to affect the fate of the cells. And lastly, it affects proliferation by means of regulating other pathways such as the Hippo pathway. But a number of questions remain unanswered about the precise nature of the crosstalk between polarity and proliferation. Distinguishing direct from indirect effects remains a big challenge, and the evidence for direct interactions is scarce. Are these processes co-ordinated or truly linked mechanistically? For example, during mouse cortical development, both overexpression of apical polarity determinants (PAR-3 and PAR-6) and shortening of G_1- phase (by cyclin D/CDK4 overexpression) expand progenitors by increasing their symmetric proliferation divisions. Whether polarity components modulate molecules regulating the G_1- phase of the cell cycle directly remains to be addressed.

Perhaps some mechanistic clues can be provided from studies of the cell cycle in non-polarized systems, such as cells in culture. For example, in a non-polarized cell culture system, aPKC has been shown to directly phosphorylate and destabilize the CIP (CDK-interacting protein)/KIP (kinase inhibitory protein) family member of cell-cycle kinase inhibitor p21^{Cip1}, in an insulin-dependent manner, linking energy metabolism and the cell cycle [51]. A similar kind of destabilization of p27^{Kip1}, another negative regulator of the cell cycle, was observed when aPKC regulated the oestrogen-induced nuclear transport of ERK (extracellular-signal-regulated kinase) 2 [52]. Studies on lung cancer using human alveolar adenocarcinoma cells in culture have also shown that aPKCι functions as an oncogene and transforms the cells via Rac1 activation, leading to the ERK1/2 signalling downstream of it [53,54]. aPKC also directly phosphorylates and stabilizes Src-3 (steroid receptor activator 3), a known oncogene and a regulator of cell proliferation. This causes transcriptional up-regulation of c-Myc and cyclin D1, promoting cellular growth and the cell cycle [55]. Thus aPKC feeds directly into the cell-cycle machinery, both at transcriptional and post-transcriptional levels, and enhances cell proliferation; however, whether this holds true in the case of cell cycle of polarized epithelium remains to be addressed.

Apical aPKC–PAR complex seems to have a leading role in stem cell renewal. Detailing the mechanisms behind the action of this complex remains a challenge for the future. Ultimate proof that cell polarity and proliferation are linked will require a biochemical understanding of their mechanistic links. At present the intersection of the Hippo pathway with the cell cycle offers the most promise in that respect. In the case of aPKC, understanding how it affects the cell cycle will require the identification of phosphorylation targets of aPKC involved in self-renewal/proliferation in any of the model systems mentioned in the present chapter.

Summary

- *Apicobasal polarity and proliferation of stem/progenitor cells are two fundamental cellular processes that are highly co-ordinated and mechanistically linked during development.*
- *While a polarized progenitor shows unlimited proliferation potential, a non-polarized progenitor tends to exit the cell cycle and differentiate.*
- *The polarization state of a cell affects the way it divides, symmetrically or asymmetrically, and this has profound effects on the cell-cycle exit properties of the daughter cells and their subsequent fate.*
- *Polarity affects the cell-cycle kinetics of cells, which itself is associated with their cell-cycle exit properties and fate.*
- *Polarity components also affect cell proliferation by means of regulating the Hippo signalling pathway, a key sensor of cell growth and cycle.*
- *The key polarity molecule promoting stem cell proliferation is aPKC, which is actively involved in all of the mechanisms described above. Identifying the phosphorylation targets of aPKC will shed light on the biochemical mechanistic details behind its action on stem cell proliferation.*

References

1. Baas, A.F., Kuipers, J., van der Wel, N.N., Batlle, E., Koerten, H.K., Peters, P.J. and Clevers, H.C. (2004) Complete polarization of single intestinal epithelial cells upon activation of LKB1 by STRAD. Cell **116**, 457–466
2. Suzuki, A. and Ohno, S. (2006) The PAR-aPKC system: lessons in polarity. J. Cell Sci. **119**, 979–987
3. Betschinger, J. and Knoblich, J.A. (2004) Dare to be different: asymmetric cell division in *Drosophila, C. elegans* and vertebrates. Curr. Biol. **14**, R674–R685
4. Collins, K., Jacks, T. and Pavletich, N.P. (1997) The cell cycle and cancer. Proc. Natl. Acad. Sci. U.S.A. **94**, 2776–2778
5. Locker, M., Agathocleous, M., Amato, M.A., Parain, K., Harris, W.A. and Perron, M. (2006) Hedgehog signaling and the retina: insights into the mechanisms controlling the proliferative properties of neural precursors. Genes Dev. **20**, 3036–3048
6. Knoblich, J.A. (2010) Asymmetric cell division: recent developments and their implications for tumour biology. Nat. Rev. **11**, 849–860
7. Spana, E.P. and Doe, C.Q. (1996) Numb antagonizes Notch signaling to specify sibling neuron cell fates. Neuron **17**, 21–26
8. Spana, E.P. and Doe, C.Q. (1995) The prospero transcription factor is asymmetrically localized to the cell cortex during neuroblast mitosis in *Drosophila*. Development **121**, 3187–3195
9. Hirata, J., Nakagoshi, H., Nabeshima, Y. and Matsuzaki, F. (1995) Asymmetric segregation of the homeodomain protein Prospero during *Drosophila* development. Nature **377**, 627–630
10. Choksi, S.P., Southall, T.D., Bossing, T., Edoff, K., de Wit, E., Fischer, B.E., van Steensel, B., Micklem, G. and Brand, A.H. (2006) Prospero acts as a binary switch between self-renewal and differentiation in *Drosophila* neural stem cells. Dev. Cell **11**, 775–789

11. Betschinger, J., Mechtler, K. and Knoblich, J.A. (2006) Asymmetric segregation of the tumor suppressor brat regulates self-renewal in *Drosophila* neural stem cells. Cell **124**, 1241–1253

12. Bilder, D. (2004) Epithelial polarity and proliferation control: links from the *Drosophila* neoplastic tumor suppressors. Genes Dev. **18**, 1909–1925

13. Gotz, M. and Huttner, W.B. (2005) The cell biology of neurogenesis. Nat. Rev. **6**, 777–788

14. Cappello, S., Attardo, A., Wu, X., Iwasato, T., Itohara, S., Wilsch-Brauninger, M., Eilken, H.M., Rieger, M.A., Schroeder, T.T., Huttner, W.B. et al. (2006) The Rho-GTPase cdc42 regulates neural progenitor fate at the apical surface. Nat. Neurosci. **9**, 1099–1107

15. Takahashi, T., Nowakowski, R.S. and Caviness, Jr, V.S. (1995) The cell cycle of the pseudostratified ventricular epithelium of the embryonic murine cerebral wall. J. Neurosci. **15**, 6046–6057

16. Arai, Y., Pulvers, J.N., Haffner, C., Schilling, B., Nusslein, I., Calegari, F., Huttner, W.B. (2011) Neural stem and progenitor cells shorten S-phase on commitment to neuron production. Nat. Commun. **2**, 154

17. Pilaz, L.J., Patti, D., Marcy, G., Ollier, E., Pfister, S., Douglas, R.J., Betizeau, M., Gautier, E., Cortay, V., Doerflinger, N. et al. (2009) Forced G1-phase reduction alters mode of division, neuron number, and laminar phenotype in the cerebral cortex. Proc. Natl. Acad. Sci. U.S.A. **106**, 21924–21929

18. Lange, C., Huttner, W.B. and Calegari, F. (2009) Cdk4/cyclinD1 overexpression in neural stem cells shortens G1, delays neurogenesis, and promotes the generation and expansion of basal progenitors. Cell Stem Cell **5**, 320–331

19. Lange, C. and Calegari, F. (2010) Cdks and cyclins link G1 length and differentiation of embryonic, neural and hematopoietic stem cells. Cell Cycle **9**, 1893–1900

20. Chalmers, A.D., Pambos, M., Mason, J., Lang, S., Wylie, C. and Papalopulu, N. (2005) aPKC, Crumbs3 and Lgl2 control apicobasal polarity in early vertebrate development. Development **132**, 977–986

21. Chalmers, A.D., Welchman, D. and Papalopulu, N. (2002) Intrinsic differences between the superficial and deep layers of the *Xenopus* ectoderm control primary neuronal differentiation. Dev. Cell **2**, 171–182

22. Lee, M. and Vasioukhin, V. (2008) Cell polarity and cancer: cell and tissue polarity as a non-canonical tumor suppressor. J. Cell Sci. **121**, 1141–1150

23. Gateff, E. (1978) Malignant neoplasms of genetic origin in *Drosophila melanogaster*. Science **200**, 1448–1459

24. Bilder, D., Li, M. and Perrimon, N. (2000) Cooperative regulation of cell polarity and growth by *Drosophila* tumor suppressors. Science **289**, 113–116

25. Wodarz, A. and Nathke, I. (2007) Cell polarity in development and cancer. Nat. Cell Biol. **9**, 1016–1024

26. Genevet, A. and Tapon, N. The Hippo pathway and apico-basal cell polarity. Biochem. J. **436**, 213–224

27. Lee, C.Y., Andersen, R.O., Cabernard, C., Manning, L., Tran, K.D., Lanskey, M.J., Bashirullah, A. and Doe, C.Q. (2006) *Drosophila* Aurora-A kinase inhibits neuroblast self-renewal by regulating aPKC/Numb cortical polarity and spindle orientation. Genes Dev. **20**, 3464–3474

28. Rolls, M.M., Albertson, R., Shih, H.P., Lee, C.Y. and Doe, C.Q. (2003) *Drosophila* aPKC regulates cell polarity and cell proliferation in neuroblasts and epithelia. J. Cell Biol. **163**, 1089–1098

29. Betschinger, J., Mechtler, K. and Knoblich, J.A. (2003) The Par complex directs asymmetric cell division by phosphorylating the cytoskeletal protein Lgl. Nature **422**, 326–330

30. Atwood, S.X. and Prehoda, K.E. (2009) aPKC phosphorylates Miranda to polarize fate determinants during neuroblast asymmetric cell division. Curr Biol. **19**, 723–729

31. Smith, C.A., Lau, K.M., Rahmani, Z., Dho, S.E., Brothers, G., She, Y.M., Berry, D.M., Bonneil, E., Thibault, P., Schweisguth, F. et al. (2007) aPKC-mediated phosphorylation regulates asymmetric membrane localization of the cell fate determinant Numb. EMBO J. **26**, 468–480

32. Wodarz, A., Ramrath, A., Grimm, A. and Knust, E. (2000) *Drosophila* atypical protein kinase C associates with Bazooka and controls polarity of epithelia and neuroblasts. J. Cell Biol. **150**, 1361–1374

33. Lee, C.Y., Robinson, K.J. and Doe, C.Q. (2006) Lgl, Pins and aPKC regulate neuroblast self-renewal versus differentiation. Nature **439**, 594–598
34. Chabu, C. and Doe, C.Q. (2008) Dap160/intersectin binds and activates aPKC to regulate cell polarity and cell cycle progression. Development **135**, 2739–2746
35. Chabu, C. and Doe, C.Q. (2009) Twins/PP2A regulates aPKC to control neuroblast cell polarity and self-renewal. Dev. Biol. **330**, 399–405
36. Cabernard, C. and Doe, C.Q. (2009) Apical/basal spindle orientation is required for neuroblast homeostasis and neuronal differentiation in *Drosophila*. Dev. Cell **17**, 134–141
37. Brumby, A., Secombe, J., Horsfield, J., Coombe, M., Amin, N., Coates, D., Saint, R. and Richardson, H. (2004) A genetic screen for dominant modifiers of a cyclin E hypomorphic mutation identifies novel regulators of S-phase entry in *Drosophila*. Genetics **168**, 227–251
38. Grzeschik, N.A., Parsons, L.M., Allott, M.L., Harvey, K.F., Richardson, H.E. (2010) Lgl, aPKC, and Crumbs regulate the Salvador/Warts/Hippo pathway through two distinct mechanisms. Curr. Biol. **20**, 573–581
39. Ho, L.L., Wei, X., Shimizu, T., Lai, Z.C. (2010) Mob as tumor suppressor is activated at the cell membrane to control tissue growth and organ size in *Drosophila*. Dev. Biol. **337**, 274–283
40. Pan, D. (2010) The hippo signaling pathway in development and cancer. Dev. Cell **19**, 491–505
41. Buther, K., Plaas, C., Barnekow, A. and Kremerskothen, J. (2004) KIBRA is a novel substrate for protein kinase Cζ. Biochem. Biophys. Res. Commun. **317**, 703–707
42. Chen, C.L., Gajewski, K.M., Hamaratoglu, F., Bossuyt, W., Sansores-Garcia, L., Tao, C. and Halder, G. (2010) The apical-basal cell polarity determinant Crumbs regulates Hippo signaling in *Drosophila*. Proc. Natl. Acad. Sci. U.S.A. **107**, 15810–15815
43. Ling, C., Zheng, Y., Yin, F., Yu, J., Huang, J., Hong, Y., Wu, S. and Pan, D. (2010) The apical transmembrane protein Crumbs functions as a tumor suppressor that regulates Hippo signaling by binding to Expanded. Proc. Natl. Acad. Sci. U.S.A. **107**, 10532–10537
44. Grzeschik, N.A., Amin, N., Secombe, J., Brumby, A.M. and Richardson, H.E. (2007) Abnormalities in cell proliferation and apico-basal cell polarity are separable in *Drosophila* lgl mutant clones in the developing eye. Dev. Biol. **311**, 106–123
45. Parsons, L.M., Grzeschik, N.A., Allott, M.L. and Richardson, H.E. (2010 Lgl/aPKC and Crb regulate the Salvador/Warts/Hippo pathway. Fly **4**, 288–293
46. Alessi, D.R., Sakamoto, K. and Bayascas, J.R. (2006) LKB1-dependent signaling pathways. Annu. Rev. Biochem. **75**, 137–163
47. Hough, C.D., Woods, D.F., Park, S. and Bryant, P.J. (1997) Organizing a functional junctional complex requires specific domains of the *Drosophila* MAGUK Discs large. Genes Dev. **11**, 3242–3253
48. Costa, M.R., Wen, G., Lepier, A., Schroeder, T. and Gotz, M. (2008) Par-complex proteins promote proliferative progenitor divisions in the developing mouse cerebral cortex. Development **135**, 11–22
49. Sabherwal, N., Tsutsui, A., Hodge, S., Wei, J., Chalmers, A.D. and Papalopulu, N. (2009) The apicobasal polarity kinase aPKC functions as a nuclear determinant and regulates cell proliferation and fate during *Xenopus* primary neurogenesis. Development **136**, 2767–2777
50. Tabler, J.M., Yamanaka, H. and Green, J.B. (2010) PAR-1 promotes primary neurogenesis and asymmetric cell divisions via control of spindle orientation. Development **137**, 2501–2505
51. Scott, M.T., Ingram, A. and Ball, K.L. (2002) PDK1-dependent activation of atypical PKC leads to degradation of the p21 tumour modifier protein. EMBO J. **21**, 6771–6780
52. Castoria, G., Migliaccio, A., Di Domenico, M., Lombardi, M., de Falco, A., Varricchio, L., Bilancio, A., Barone, M.V. and Auricchio, F. (2004) Role of atypical protein kinase C in estradiol-triggered G1/S progression of MCF-7 cells. Mol. Cell. Biol. **24**, 7643–7653
53. Regala, R.P., Weems, C., Jamieson, L., Copland, J.A., Thompson, E.A. and Fields, A.P. (2005) Atypical protein kinase Cι plays a critical role in human lung cancer cell growth and tumorigenicity. J. Biol. Chem. **280**, 31109–31115

54. Regala, R.P., Weems, C., Jamieson, L., Khoor, A., Edell, E.S., Lohse, C.M. and Fields, A.P. (2005) Atypical protein kinase Cι is an oncogene in human non-small cell lung cancer. Cancer Res. **65**, 8905–8911

55. Yi, P., Feng, Q., Amazit, L., Lonard, D.M., Tsai, S.Y., Tsai, M.J. and O'Malley, B.W. (2008) Atypical protein kinase C regulates dual pathways for degradation of the oncogenic coactivator SRC-3/AIB1. Mol. Cell **29**, 465–476

© The Authors Journal compilation © 2012 Biochemical Society
Essays Biochem. (2012) **53**, 111–127: doi: 10.1042/BSE0530111

9

The Hippo pathway: key interaction and catalytic domains in organ growth control, stem cell self-renewal and tissue regeneration

Claire Cherrett, Makoto Furutani-Seiki and Stefan Bagby[1]

Department of Biology and Biochemistry, University of Bath, Bath BA2 7AY, U.K.

Abstract

The Hippo pathway is a conserved pathway that interconnects with several other pathways to regulate organ growth, tissue homoeostasis and regeneration, and stem cell self-renewal. This pathway is unique in its capacity to orchestrate multiple processes, from sensing to execution, necessary for organ expansion. Activation of the Hippo pathway core kinase cassette leads to cytoplasmic sequestration of the nuclear effectors YAP (Yes-associated protein) and TAZ (transcriptional coactivator with PDZ-binding motif), consequently disabling their transcriptional co-activation function. Components upstream of the core kinase cassette have not been well understood, especially in vertebrates, but are gradually being elucidated and include cell polarity and cell adhesion proteins.

[1]To whom correspondence should be addressed (email s.bagby@bath.ac.uk).

Introduction

Like many signalling proteins, Hippo pathway proteins are modular and use various interaction and catalytic domains to transmit signals and regulate transcription of target genes, often in a context-dependent fashion. In the present chapter we outline the major protein components, and focus on the structure and function of some of the key Hippo pathway domains in vertebrates.

The Hippo pathway and its role in organ growth control

The Hippo pathway has emerged over the last decade as a key player in organ size regulation during development, tissue homoeostasis throughout adult life, tissue regeneration and stem cell self-renewal [1–8]. Perhaps unsurprisingly, the pathway also plays a role in tumour suppression. Hippo pathway components were first identified through loss-of-function genetic screens in *Drosophila melanogaster*; the *Hpo* gene, after which the pathway has been called, was named for the mutant overgrown head phenotype that resembled hippopotamus hide [9].

Hippo pathway components

The core elements of the Hippo pathway are well known, but additional components constituting an extended network continue to be identified. Core components of the vertebrate pathway (Figure 1) include the MST [mammalian Ste (sterile) 20-like] 1/2 kinases, each of which autophosphorylates its activation loop, and then phosphorylates and forms an active complex with Sav1. MST1/2 can then phosphorylate the LATS (large tumour suppressor) 1/2 kinases and their co-activator MOB1 (Mps one binder). LATS1 or LATS2 subsequently phosphorylate the most downstream targets of the Hippo pathway, YAP (Yes-associated protein) and TAZ (transcriptional coactivator with PDZ-binding motif), enabling 14-3-3 proteins to bind and sequester YAP/TAZ in the cytoplasm (Figure 1). The Hippo pathway is less complex in *Drosophila* than in vertebrates; where two orthologues exist in vertebrates, for example, only one exists in *Drosophila*. The core components in *Drosophila*, with vertebrate homologues in parentheses, are Hippo (MST1/2), Sav (Sav1), Warts (LATS1/2), MATS (MOB1) and Yorkie (YAP/TAZ).

When the Hippo pathway is inactivated, YAP and TAZ translocate to the nucleus where they behave as co-activators for various transcription factors. YAP and TAZ lack a DBD (DNA-binding domain) and so influence transcription by interacting with DNA-binding proteins. Organ growth is promoted by the interaction of YAP and TAZ with TEAD family transcription factors which up-regulate transcription of genes that promote cell proliferation, survival, differentiation and morphogenesis [10]. TEAD transcription factors are ubiquitously expressed, although each TEAD protein (TEAD1–TEAD4) occupies a slightly different niche with respect to tissue expression and developmental stage.

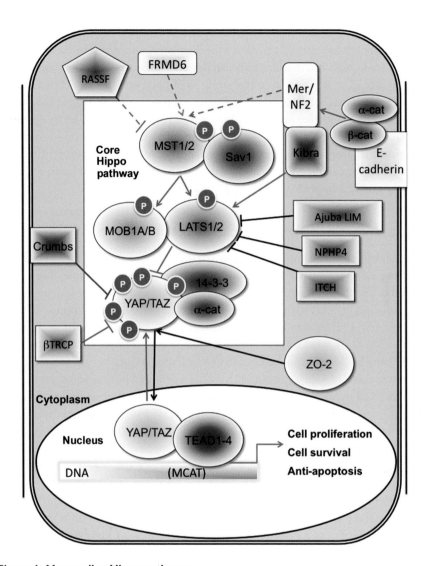

Figure 1. Mammalian Hippo pathway
The core Hippo pathway components within the orange-bordered box (MST1/2 kinases, scaffolding protein Sav1, LATS1/2 kinases and their co-factors MOB1A/B) target transcriptional co-activator proteins YAP and TAZ for phosphorylation. Phosphorylated YAP and TAZ are subsequently anchored in the cytoplasm by 14-3-3 proteins and the interaction is stabilized by α-catenin. Molecules coloured in grey antagonize the Hippo pathway by inhibiting the core kinases. Inactivation of the Hippo pathway allows YAP and TAZ to translocate into the nucleus where they contribute to the up-regulation of target genes through interactions with transcription factors.

Knowledge of upstream signals that regulate organ size and morphology is key to understanding and modulating the Hippo pathway. Recent studies have highlighted the influence of cell contacts on regulation of Hippo and associated pathways. The Crb (Crumbs) complex, which is associated with tight junctions in the sub-apical region of the cell membrane, regulates the Hippo pathway in

Drosophila through interactions with the upstream Hippo regulator Ex (Expanded) [11]. It is unclear whether the Crb–Ex mechanism is conserved in mammals but, in response to high cell density, Crb can directly inhibit nuclear translocation of YAP (Figure 1), in addition to contributing to Hippo pathway activation through an unidentified mechanism [12]. E-cadherin, a transmembrane protein that forms the intercellular epithelial junction complex, was recently found to be an upstream regulator of the Hippo pathway. E-cadherin induces cell contact inhibition, a phenomenon that stops cellular proliferation upon confluence. E-cadherin recruits β-catenin to the cell membrane, and β-catenin then activates the Hippo pathway through interactions with Merlin/NF2 (neurofibromin 2) [13].

Organ growth control and tumorigenesis

Hippo signalling orchestrates organ growth through its co-ordination of cell proliferation, survival, differentiation and polarity. Numerous examples have illustrated that deregulation of the pathway leads to significantly increased organ size. Up-regulation of YAP, the target protein that is inhibited by the Hippo pathway, increased mouse liver size from approximately 5% of body weight to approximately 25% in 4 weeks [14]. Similarly, when core Hippo pathway proteins MST1/2 and Sav1 were knocked out in mouse livers, the organs were significantly larger than those of wild-type mice [15–18]. An enlarged heart phenotype has also been observed in Sav1-knockout mice [19]. In all cases, organ structure was preserved, as observed previously for *Drosophila* Hippo pathway mutants which also display enlarged organs (heads, imaginal discs) with normal tissue patterns [20].

Constitutive YAP overexpression or liver-specific deletion of MST1/2 or Sav1 induces multi-focal tumorigenesis, highlighting the role of the pathway in tumour suppression [14,16–18]. YAP and TAZ can induce anchorage-independent growth and EMT (epithelial–mesenchymal transition) of immortalized mammary and pancreatic epithelial cells [12]. EMT is important in normal morphological processes, but when deregulated in cancers is involved in metastasis, tumour recurrence and therapeutic resistance. Upstream Hippo pathway components function as tumour suppressors. Hippo pathway mutations have been observed in a range of human cancers, including breast cancers, soft tissue sarcomas, melanomas, colorectal cancers, ovarian carcinomas, retinoblastomas, astrocytomas and neurofibromatosis type 2 [1,5]. There has been speculation about the possible involvement of Hippo signalling in cancer stem cells due to the link of the pathway to stem cell self-renewal and cancer; recently the Hippo pathway, via TAZ, was identified as a molecular link between EMT, cell polarity and cancer stem cells in breast cancer [21].

Integration of multi-pathway signalling

The Hippo pathway interacts with numerous other signalling pathways (Table 1), some of which contribute to organ growth regulation. This cross-talk occurs in both cytoplasm and nucleus, and is probably important for the tight control of cell proliferation, growth, polarity and differentiation required for formation and maintenance of functional proportionate organs without crossing the boundary into tumorigenesis. Some of the inter-connections with the Hippo pathway are described below [2,7,8,22].

Canonical Wnt pathway

Wnt signalling activates membrane-bound Dvl (Dishevelled) which inhibits the axin–GSK (glycogen synthase kinase) 3–APC (adenomatous polyposis coli) β-catenin destruction complex (β-catenin is the nuclear effector of Wnt

Table 1. Cross-talk between Hippo pathway proteins and other signalling pathways

EGFR, epidermal growth factor receptor; FOXO, forkhead box O; JAK, Janus kinase; PI3K, phosphoinositide 3-kinase; Rb, retinoblastoma; Shh, Sonic hedgehog; STAT, signal transducer and activator of transcription.

Pathway cross-talk	Hippo pathway protein interaction
The Hippo pathway inhibits Wnt/β-catenin signalling [23]	Direct interaction of TAZ with Dvl2 inhibits phosphorylation of Dvl2 by CK1δ/ε thereby preventing formation of the β-catenin destruction complex. This results in β-catenin nuclear localization and expression of Wnt target genes.
The Hippo pathway inhibits BMP/TGFβ signalling [12,44]	Direct interaction of YAP with phospho-Smad1 and YAP/TAZ with phospho-Smad2/3 retains Smads in the nucleus and leads to transcription of TGFβ/Smad target genes.
The Hippo pathway inhibits JAK/STAT signalling [45]	Nuclear Yki induces transcription of cytokines that promote JAK/STAT signalling in response to injury.
The Hippo pathway inhibits Notch signalling [46]	Nuclear Yki inhibits the Notch ligand Delta which leads to Notch activation.
Shh signalling inhibits the Hippo pathway [47]	Shh signalling up-regulates expression of YAP1 mRNA, and stabilizes IRS1 (insulin receptor substrate 1) which acts as a nuclear retention factor for YAP. Shh signalling also results in decreased levels of phospho-LATS.
The Hippo pathway promotes FOXO signalling [48]	MST1 phosphorylates FOXO proteins leading to nuclear localization and transcription of FOXO target genes.
PI3K/Akt signalling inhibits the Hippo pathway [49]	Akt phosphorylates MST1 (at Thr^{120}), thereby preventing the kinase activity of MST1.
Rb [50,51]	The transcription factor E2F is negatively regulated by Rb. E2F interacts with the Yki–Sd complex and therefore Rb inhibits E2F–Yki–Sd mediated transcription. In humans, LATS phosphorylates DYRK (dual-specificity tyrosine phosphorylation-regulated kinase) which leads to activation of the 'DREAM' complex and inhibition of E2F.
EGFR signalling [52]	YAP mediates transcription of the EGFR ligand amphiregulin, leading to proliferation and migration of neighbouring cells.

signalling). When membrane-localized β-catenin dissociates from E-cadherin and α-catenin, it translocates to the nucleus where it interacts with Lef (lymphoid enhancer factor)/TCF (T-cell factor) transcription factors, causing the activation of target genes that determine stem cell survival and differentiation. The Hippo pathway inhibits the canonical Wnt pathway by enhancing levels of cytoplasmic phosphorylated TAZ, which binds to Dvl [23]. This interaction prevents phosphorylation of Dvl, rendering Dvl inactive. In the absence of hyperphosphorylated Dvl, β-catenin does not reach the nucleus and is targeted for degradation. The links between Hippo and Wnt signalling are not limited to the cytoplasmic TAZ–Dvl interaction; the E-cadherin–β-catenin–α-catenin complex binds Merlin and activates the Hippo pathway [13]. Also, upon Hippo pathway abrogation, nuclear non-phosphorylated TEAD-bound YAP forms a complex with Lef/TCF-bound β-catenin. YAP–β-catenin complex formation leads to up-regulation of *Sox2* and *Snai2* genes, and a consequent increase in heart size [19].

TGFβ (transforming growth factor β) and BMP (bone morphogenetic protein) signalling

The Hippo pathway has multiple connections with TGFβ and BMP signalling. Upon TGFβ or BMP interaction with their respective membrane-bound receptors, cytoplasmic Smad proteins are activated by phosphorylation in the C-terminal region. Smad proteins contain an N-terminal MH1 domain that binds DNA and a C-terminal MH2 protein–protein interaction domain. Upon activation, Smads translocate to the nucleus where they form transcription factor complexes. When nuclear Smad2/3 forms a complex with nuclear YAP/TAZ, Smad2/3 is prevented from returning to the cytoplasm and genes that promote EMT are up-regulated [12]. Phosphorylation of the Smad inter-MH domain linker by CDK (cyclin-dependent kinase) 8/9 promotes the Smad–YAP/TAZ interaction which up-regulates transcription of target genes when the proteins are nuclear [24]. The Hippo pathway can therefore inhibit TGFβ and BMP signalling by inducing cytoplasmic retention of YAP/TAZ, consequently sequestering YAP/TAZ-bound Smad2/3 or Smad1/5/8 proteins to the cytoplasm.

Mechanotransduction

An increase in ECM (extracellular matrix) rigidity, such as in bone, causes Rho GTPase activation and leads to stress fibre formation. When cytoskeletal tension increases in response to stiff ECM, YAP and TAZ are retained within the nucleus and MSCs (mesenchymal stem cells) differentiate into osteoblasts. Conversely, when the MSCs are grown on soft ECM with low intracellular cytoskeletal tension, YAP and TAZ are excluded from the nucleus, and the cells can differentiate into other lineages, such as adipocytes. The Hippo pathway regulator E-cadherin can control Rho activation, but in this case E-cadherin may not be involved as mechanotransduction-mediated control of YAP/TAZ cellular localization occurs independently of the core Hippo pathway [25].

Pro-apoptotic and other interactions

In addition to TEADs and Smads, YAP and TAZ interact with other transcription factors, for example PPARγ (peroxisome-proliferator-activated receptor γ) and p73, which can result in repressed transcription or pro-apoptotic effects. YAP and TAZ interact with a host of other proteins (Table 2), in some cases without any apparent connection to the canonical Hippo pathway. As YAP and TAZ are the most downstream targets of the pathway, elucidating the function of these YAP/TAZ complexes is vital for understanding the control of organogenesis and tissue homoeostasis.

Table 2. Binding partners of YAP and TAZ

Binding protein	Description of binding protein	YAP/TAZ domain involved
14-3-3 [53,54]	Dimeric proteins that sequester YAP/TAZ to the cytoplasm	Phosphorylated 14-3-3-binding motif
AMOT [55]	Angiomotin, part of the Crumbs complex	WW domain(s)
ASPP1/2 (p53BP) [56]	Apoptosis-stimulating protein of p53 protein family	WW domain(s)
c-Yes [57]	Tyrosine kinase	SH3-binding motif
Crb [12]	Upstream Hippo pathway complex protein Crumbs	WW domain(s) and PDZ-binding motif
Dvl2 [23]	Dishevelled polarity protein involved in Wnt signalling	WW domain and PDZ-binding motif
ErbB4 [58]	Receptor tyrosine kinase that contains a cleavable cytoplasmic fragment	WW domain(s)
Ex [59]	Upstream Hippo pathway FERM-domain protein	WW domain(s)
HNRNPU [60]	Heterogenous nuclear ribonuclear protein U binds to YAP and p73	Proline-rich region at N-terminus of YAP
LATS1/2 [61,62]	Hippo pathway serine/threonine kinases	WW domain(s)
NFE2 (p45) [63]	Haemopoietic transcription factor-2	WW domain(s)
NHERF (EPB50) [53,64]	Recruits YAP and TAZ to plasma membrane	PDZ-binding motif
p73 [65,66]	Pro-apoptotic transcription factor	WW domain(s)
PEBP2 [31]	Polyoma enhancer binding protein 2 transcription factor	WW domain(s)
PPARγ [67]	Adipocyte transcription factor	WW domain(s)
PRGP2 [68]	Proline-rich membrane Gla protein	WW domain(s)
Runx1/2 [67,69]	Transcription factors with Runt DNA-binding domain	WW domain(s)
Smads [24,44]	Transcription factors regulated by the TGFβ BMP signalling pathway	WW domain(s)
TEAD [70]	Transcription factors	TBD
WBP1/2 [71]	WW domain-binding proteins	WW domain(s)

Key Hippo pathway domains

Regulation of organ growth, tissue homoeostasis, tissue regeneration and stem cell self-renewal by Hippo pathway components depends on protein–protein, protein–nucleic acid and protein–membrane interactions, and in some instances multi-protein complex formation. The binding properties of a range of domains or motifs within Hippo pathway proteins promote these interactions. Hippo pathway proteins generally contain multiple domains or motifs separated by various lengths of often unstructured polypeptide (Figure 2).

TEAD–YAP/TAZ interaction domains

The major nuclear proteins regulated by the Hippo pathway are the TEAD transcription factors (Figure 1). TEAD proteins comprise an N-terminal DBD and a C-terminal YBD (YAP-binding domain), both of which are indispensable because individually YAP and TEAD have no transcriptional activity. The TEAD DBD can bind to a variety of M-CAT-like DNA sequences (the M-CAT motif is 5'-TCATTCCT-3') in a fairly promiscuous manner. The solution structure of the human TEAD1 (TEF-1) A49S mutant DBD comprises a three-helix bundle in a homeodomain-like fold. The first two α-helices are almost anti-parallel with the third α-helix lying across them (Figure 3). Similar to homeodomain proteins, DNA binding is mediated by the third α-helix (H3) and the preceding loop (L2); H1 and L1 do not bind directly, but are necessary for full-strength binding of TEAD to tandem M-CAT sites [26].

   The TBD (TEAD-binding domain) of YAP/TAZ, located in the N-terminal region, is natively unstructured and binds TEAD with high fidelity – to date no other protein interactions are known to involve the TBD. The crystal structures of YAP–TEAD interaction domains involving human TEAD2 [27], human TEAD1–YAP [28] and mouse TEAD4–YAP [29] show that the TEAD YBDs adopt an immunoglobulin-like β-sandwich fold with the addition of two helix-turn-helix motifs (Figure 3). The Y421H mutation in TEAD1 that is present in human Sveinsson's chorioretinal atrophy was previously found to abrogate interactions with YAP and TAZ [30]. Consistent with this, Tyr[421] is located in the TEAD–YAP interface where it forms a hydrogen bond with a serine residue in YAP (Ser[94] in human YAP). Upon interaction with TEAD, the YAP TBD forms two α-helices that pack into binding grooves and are separated by an extended loop that wraps around the YBD [28,29].

YAP/TAZ TAD (transcription activation domain)

Both YAP and TAZ contain a C-terminal TAD [31]. Although there have been no experimental studies of the structure of this domain, secondary structure predictions indicate that it is largely unstructured.

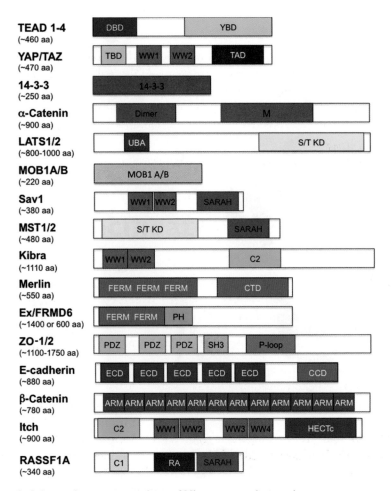

Figure 2. Schematic representations of Hippo network proteins

aa, amino acid; DBD, DNA-binding domain; YBD, YAP-binding domain; TBD, TEAD-binding domain; WW, domain containing two signature tryptophan residues; TAD, transactivation domain; M, vinculin-like domain; UBA, ubiquitin-associated domain; S/T KD, serine/threonine kinase domain; SARAH, Sav/Rassf/Hippo domain; FERM, 4.1 protein/ezrin/radixin/moesin domain; CTD, C-terminal domain; PH, pleckstrin homology domain; PDZ, PSD-95 (postsynaptic density 95), Dlg (discs large) and zonula occludens-1 domain; SH3, Src homology 3 domain; P-loop, NTPase domain; ECD, extracellular cadherin domain; CCD, cytoplasmic cadherin domain; ARM, armadillo repeat; HECTc, homologous with E6-associated protein C-terminus; RA, Ras-association domain.

YAP/TAZ cytoplasmic sequestration by 14-3-3

C-terminal to the YAP/TAZ TBD is an HxRxxS motif that becomes a 14-3-3-binding site upon serine phosphorylation (Ser[127] in human YAP). A crystal structure of the homodimeric 14-3-3σ–YAP phospho-peptide complex (Figure 3) reveals that the YAP peptide binds to each monomer of 14-3-3σ with

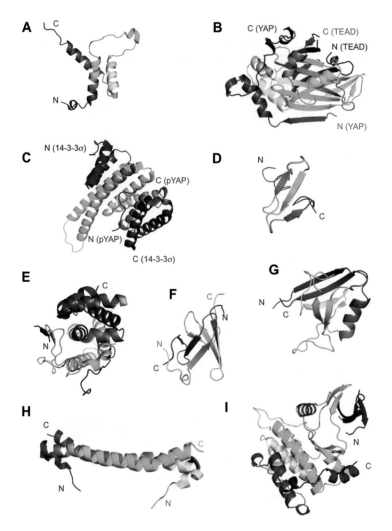

Figure 3. Structures of some Hippo pathway protein domains
(**A**), (**D**), (**F**) and (**H**) are NMR solution structures; (**B**), (**C**), (**E**), (**G**) and (**I**) are crystal structures. (**A**) TEAD1 DBD (PDB ID: 2HZD); (**B**) TEAD1 YBD–YAP TBD complex (PDB ID: 3KYS); (**C**) 14-3-3σ–YAP phospho-peptide complex (PDB ID: 3MHR); (**D**) YAP WW2 domain (PDB ID: 2L4J); (**E**) S. cerevisiae MOB1 (PDB ID: 2HJN); (**F**) mouse Sav WW2 domain dimer (PDB ID: 2DWV); (**G**) ZO1 PDZ1 domain (PDB ID: 2H3M); (**H**) MST1 SARAH domain (PDB ID: 2JO8); and (**I**) MST1 kinase domain (PDB ID: 3COM).

a 1:1 stoichiometry, so each 14-3-3 dimer can bind two molecules of YAP [32]. 14-3-3σ dimerizes in a W-shape via α-helices 1–4. Helices 3, 5, 7 and 9 on each monomer form the YAP-binding groove. The YAP peptide-bound 14-3-3σ structure is very similar to unbound 14-3-3σ with an overall r.m.s.d. (root mean square deviation) between the structures of 1.00 Å (1 Å = 0.1 nm), suggesting that YAP binding does not induce a large conformational change in 14-3-3.

WW domains

WW domains are prevalent and important features of the Hippo pathway: YAP, TAZ, Sav1, Kibra and Itch each contain at least one WW domain [33]. The WW domain (approximately 40 residues) is the smallest known protein domain and consists of a twisted three-stranded β-sheet (Figure 3). WW domains are named after two signature tryptophan residues located on the first and third β-strands. The first tryptophan residue is required for folding and the second tryptophan residue is involved in ligand binding [34]. WW domains are central mediators of protein binding events throughout the extended Hippo network via interactions with proline-rich motifs. WW domains are categorized into five groups (I–V) according to their cognate ligand. The main Hippo pathway WW domains fall into group I, i.e. the WW domains bind to PY motifs (PPxY and, less frequently, LPxY); such motifs are found, for example, in LATS1/2, most of the Smads, Dvl and p73.

Itch contains four WW domains and inhibits the Hippo pathway by binding to PPxY motifs of LATS1/2, predominantly via its first WW domain, leading to ubiquitination and degradation of LATS1/2 [35]. Sav1 and Kibra both contain two WW domains; in each case, WW1 is a group I domain, and WW2 is atypical in that the second tryptophan residue is replaced by another amino acid (isoleucine in Kibra, tyrosine in vertebrate Sav1 and arginine in *Drosophila* Sav). Mouse Sav1 WW2 is the only WW domain known to date to dimerize (Figure 3) [36]. Sav1 promotes multi-protein complex formation in the Hippo pathway by acting as a scaffold protein through SARAH domain multimerization. It is possible that WW2 homodimerization enhances this scaffolding function, whereas WW1 engages binding partners.

The YAP1 and YAP2 isoforms of YAP contain one and two WW domains respectively. It is not currently clear what specific roles the different isoforms play. YAP and TAZ have approximately 20 known binding partners (Table 2), many of which bind via at least one of the WW domains; given the prevalence of PPxY motifs in proteomes, the number of protein–protein interactions mediated by YAP and TAZ could be much higher than this. The WW domains of YAP and TAZ belong to group I [37], but YAP WW1 has also been found to interact with a phospho-serine motif of Smad1 [24]: phosphorylation by CDK8/9 [as part of BMP (bone morphogenetic protein) signalling] creates a YAP WW1-binding site on the Smad1 inter-MH domain linker (see above). This region also contains a PPxY motif that binds to YAP WW2. CDK8/9 phosphorylation also primes Smad1 for phosphorylation by GSK3. Secondary phosphorylation of Smad1 by GSK3 reduces the affinity for YAP WW1 and increases the affinity for Smurf1 WW1; Smurf1 WW2 simultaneously binds the PPxY motif. Interactions with Smurf1 lead to poly-ubiquitination and subsequent proteasomal degradation of Smad1, thereby marking the end of a YAP–Smad transcriptional event. Wnt signalling suppresses GSK3, providing another illustration of the complexity of interpathway connections.

SARAH domains

The SARAH coiled-coil domain is present in the C-terminal region of Sav1, Rassf and Hippo (MST1/2). SARAH domains homodimerize and can also mediate heterodimerization of Hippo pathway proteins, for example between MST1/2 and Sav1. The solution structure of the human MST1 SARAH homodimer (Figure 3) shows that each monomer comprises a short N-terminal α-helix that is oriented towards the N-terminal helix of the other monomer, and an elongated C-terminal α-helix along which the anti-parallel dimer interface lies [38]. The Rassf5 (Nore1) SARAH domain forms a homotetramer but, in the presence of the MST1 SARAH domain, only dimers are observed. The role of mammalian Rassf proteins in the Hippo pathway is currently unclear; *in vitro* studies indicate that Rassf1 and Rassf5 inhibit the Hippo pathway, as is the case for *Drosophila* Rassf. Conversely, in some cases the Hippo pathway seems to be activated by Rassf proteins *in vivo* [1].

Serine/threonine kinase domains

Central to the Hippo pathway are the serine/threonine kinase domains of MST1/2 and LATS1/2 that propagate phosphorylation events to retain YAP/TAZ in the cytoplasm. MST1/2 belong to the Ste group of kinases, whereas LATS kinases are similar to the PKC (protein kinase C) family. In a crystal structure of activated MST1 (Figure 3), the auto-activation loop is di-phosphorylated. There are currently no published structures of the LATS1 and LATS2 kinase domains.

MOB1

MOB1 is part of the MOB family of co-activator proteins [39]. Human MOB1 binding to LATS1/2 triggers LATS1/2 auto-phosphorylation on the activation segment. The MOB1–LATS1/2 complex phosphorylates YAP/TAZ. The C-terminal core domain adopts an α-helical fold common to all MOB proteins, whereas the N-terminal region is less conserved but seems to be functionally important. In *Saccharomyces cerevisiae* MOB1, this N-terminal region includes structural elements that mediate homodimerization *in vitro* [40]. One side of the MOB1 surface is mostly acidic and the opposite side is basic. Bioinformatic and experimental analyses indicate that the interaction between MOB1 and LATS1/2 is mediated by the acidic face of the former and the basic region of the N-terminal regulatory domain of the latter.

PDZ-binding motifs

YAP and TAZ contain a C-terminal PDZ-binding motif (LTWL) that allows interaction with several proteins involved in organ size regulation. PDZ domains typically comprise 80–100 residues forming six β-strands and two α-helices of differing lengths (Figure 3). The binding groove is generally located between the longer α-helix and the second β-strand [41]. Nuclear localization of YAP/TAZ is promoted by interactions with the first PDZ domain of the tight junction-associated proteins ZO (zonula occludens)-1 and -2 [42,43]. Interactions involving PDZ-binding motifs and PDZ domains, and WW domains and PPxY motifs, are important for Hippo pathway cross-talk with TGFβ signalling {YAP/TAZ interaction with Crumbs components PALS1, AMOT (angiomotin), PATJ (PALS1-associated tight junction protein) and LIN7 [12]} and with the Wnt pathway (TAZ interaction with Dvl [23]).

Other domains within Hippo pathway proteins

Remaining protein–protein interaction domains include those involved in self-association, such as the dimerization domain of α-catenin and those that lead to proteasomal degradation, e.g. the UBA (ubiquitin-associated) domain of LATS1/2. Domains involved in membrane interaction and localization include the FERM domains in Merlin and FRMD6, and the C2 domains in Kibra and Itch.

Conclusions

The Hippo pathway interconnects with numerous other pathways in order to orchestrate organ growth or tissue regeneration, and might therefore be more appropriately termed the Hippo network. Substantial knowledge of Hippo network operation has rapidly emerged, but many questions remain. In terms of protein domains, for example, how are the multiple possible WW, SARAH and PDZ domain interactions co-ordinated? What are the structural and functional relationships between multiple domains/motifs within and between proteins? How do post-translational modifications, predominantly phosphorylation, modulate domain structures and interactions? Detailed structural, biochemical, biophysical and computational analyses, including isolation or reconstitution of multimolecular complexes, are needed to answer questions such as these. In combination with cellular and organismal studies, one long-term goal of these molecular level studies is systems level comprehension of Hippo signalling towards understanding and prediction of responses to particular developmental and environmental cues, and towards controlled modulation for research and clinical applications.

Summary

- *The Hippo pathway is a central conserved pathway that interconnects with several other pathways to regulate organ growth, tissue homoeostasis and regeneration, and stem cell self-renewal.*
- *The Hippo pathway is unique in its capacity to orchestrate multiple processes, from sensing to execution, necessary for organ expansion.*
- *The mechanisms and effects of Hippo pathway cross-talk with other pathways such as Wnt and TGFβ growth factor pathways will undoubtedly turn out to be highly complex, but are gradually being elucidated.*

- *The Hippo pathway includes protein domains involved in catalysis, protein–membrane interactions, protein–protein interactions and protein–nucleic acid interactions.*

References

1. Bao, Y., Hata, Y., Ikeda, M. and Withanage, K. (2011) Mammalian Hippo pathway: from development to cancer and beyond. J. Biochem. **149**, 361–379
2. Mauviel, A., Nallet-Staub, F. and Varelas, X. (2012) Integrating developmental signals: a Hippo in the (path)way. Oncogene **31**, 1743–1756
3. Halder, G. and Johnson, R. L. (2011) Hippo signaling: growth control and beyond. Development **138**, 9–22
4. Zhao, B., Tumaneng, K. and Guan, K. L. (2011) The Hippo pathway in organ size control, tissue regeneration and stem cell self-renewal. Nat. Cell Biol. **13**, 877–883
5. Zhao, B., Li, L., Lei, Q. and Guan, K. L. (2010) The Hippo-YAP pathway in organ size control and tumorigenesis: an updated version. Genes Dev. **24**, 862–874
6. Staley, B.K. and Irvine, K.D. (2012) Hippo signaling in *Drosophila*: recent advances and insights. Dev. Dyn. **241**, 3–15
7. Varelas, X. and Wrana, J.L. (2012) Coordinating developmental signaling: novel roles for the Hippo pathway. Trends Cell Biol. **22**, 88–96
8. Sudol, M. and Harvey, K.F. (2010) Modularity in the Hippo signalling pathway. Trends Biochem. Sci. **35**, 627–633
9. Udan, R.S., Kango-Singh, M., Nolo, R., Tao, C.Y. and Halder, G. (2003) Hippo promotes proliferation arrest and apoptosis in the Salvador/Warts pathway. Nat. Cell Biol. **5**, 914–920
10. Chen, L., Loh, P.G. and Song, H. (2010) Structural and functional insights into the TEAD-YAP complex in the Hippo signaling pathway. Prot. Cell **1**, 1073–1083
11. Parsons, L.M., Grzeschik, N.A., Allott, M.L. and Richardson, H.E. (2010) Lgl/aPKC and Crb regulate the Salvador/Warts/Hippo pathway. Fly **4**, 288–293
12. Varelas, X., Samavarchi-Tehrani, P., Narimatsu, M., Weiss, A., Cockburn, K., Larsen, B.G., Rossant, J. and Wrana, J.L. (2010) The Crumbs complex couples cell density sensing to Hippo-dependent control of the TGF-β-SMAD pathway. Dev. Cell **19**, 831–844
13. Kim, N.G., Koh, E., Chen, X. and Gumbiner, B.M. (2011) E-cadherin mediates contact inhibition of proliferation through Hippo signaling-pathway components. Proc. Natl. Acad. Sci. U.S.A. **108**, 11930–11935
14. Dong, J.X., Feldmann, G., Huang, J.B., Wu, S., Zhang, N.L., Comerford, S.A., Gayyed, M.F., Anders, R.A., Maitra, A. and Pan, D.J. (2007) Elucidation of a universal size-control mechanism in *Drosophila* and mammals. Cell **130**, 1120–1133
15. Zhou, D., Conrad, C., Xia, F., Park, J.S., Payer, B., Yin, Y., Lauwers, G.Y., Thasler, W., Lee, J.T., Avruch, J. and Bardeesy, N. (2009) Mst1 and Mst2 maintain hepatocyte quiescence and suppress hepatocellular carcinoma development through inactivation of the Yap1 oncogene. Cancer Cell **16**, 425–438
16. Lu, L., Li, Y., Kim, S.M., Bossuyt, W., Liu, P., Qiu, Q., Wang, Y., Halder, G., Finegold, M.J., Lee, J.S. and Johnson, R.L. (2010) Hippo signaling is a potent *in vivo* growth and tumor suppressor pathway in the mammalian liver. Proc. Natl. Acad. Sci. U.S.A. **107**, 1437–1442
17. Song, H., Mak, K.K., Topol, L., Yun, K., Hu, J., Garrett, L., Chen, Y., Park, O., Chang, J., Simpson, R.M. et al. (2010) Mammalian Mst1 and Mst2 kinases play essential roles in organ size control and tumor suppression. Proc. Natl. Acad. Sci. U.S.A. **107**, 1431–1436
18. Lee, K.P., Lee, J.H., Kim, T.S., Kim, T.H., Park, H.D., Byun, J.S., Kim, M.C., Jeong, W.I., Calvisi, D.F., Kim, J.M. and Lim, D.S. (2010) The Hippo-Salvador pathway restrains hepatic oval cell proliferation, liver size, and liver tumorigenesis. Proc. Natl. Acad. Sci. U.S.A. **107**, 8248–8253

19. Heallen, T., Zhang, M., Wang, J., Bonilla-Claudio, M., Klysik, E., Johnson, R.L. and Martin, J.F. (2011) Hippo pathway inhibits Wnt signaling to restrain cardiomyocyte proliferation and heart size. Science **332**, 458–461

20. Kango-Singh, M. and Singh, A. (2009) Regulation of organ size: insights from the *Drosophila* Hippo signaling pathway. Dev. Dyn. **238**, 1627–1637

21. Cordenonsi, M., Zanconato, F., Azzolin, L., Forcato, M., Rosato, A., Frasson, C., Inui, M., Montagner, M., Parenti, A.R., Poletti, A. et al. (2011) The Hippo transducer TAZ confers cancer stem cell-related traits on breast cancer cells. Cell **147**, 759–772

22. McNeill, H. and Woodgett, J.R. (2010) When pathways collide: collaboration and connivance among signalling proteins in development. Nat. Rev. Mol. Cell Biol. **11**, 404–413

23. Varelas, X., Miller, B.W., Sopko, R., Song, S.Y., Gregorieff, A., Fellouse, F.A., Sakuma, R., Pawson, T., Hunziker, W., McNeill, H., Wrana, J.L. and Attisano, L. (2010) The Hippo pathway regulates Wnt/β-Catenin signaling. Dev. Cell **18**, 579–591

24. Aragon, E., Goerner, N., Zaromytidou, A.I., Xi, Q., Escobedo, A., Massagué, J. and Macias, M.J. (2011) A Smad action turnover switch operated by WW domain readers of a phosphoserine code. Genes Dev. **25**, 1275–1288

25. Dupont, S., Morsut, L., Aragona, M., Enzo, E., Giulitti, S., Cordenonsi, M., Zanconato, F., Le Digabel, J., Forcato, M., Bicciato, S. et al. (2011) Role of YAP/TAZ in mechanotransduction. Nature **474**, 179–183

26. Anbanandam, A., Albarado, D.C., Nguyen, C.T., Halder, G., Gao, X.L. and Veeraraghavan, S. (2006) Insights into transcription enhancer factor 1 (TEF-1) activity from the solution structure of the TEA domain. Proc. Natl. Acad. Sci. U.S.A. **103**, 17225–17230

27. Tian, W., Yu, J., Tomchick, D.R., Pan, D. and Luo, X. (2010) Structural and functional analysis of the YAP-binding domain of human TEAD2. Proc. Natl. Acad. Sci. U.S.A. **107**, 7293–7298

28. Li, Z., Zhao, B., Wang, P., Chen, F., Dong, Z.H., Yang, H.R., Guan, K.L. and Xu, Y.H. (2010) Structural insights into the YAP and TEAD complex. Genes Dev. **24**, 235–240

29. Chen, L.M., Chan, S.W., Zhang, X.Q., Walsh, M., Lim, C.J., Hong, W.J. and Song, H.W. (2010) Structural basis of YAP recognition by TEAD4 in the Hippo pathway. Genes Dev. **24**, 290–300

30. Kitagawa, M. (2007) A Sveinsson's chorioretinal atrophy-associated missense mutation in mouse Tead1 affects its interaction with the co-factors YAP and TAZ. Biochem. Biophys. Res. Commun. **361**, 1022–1026

31. Yagi, R., Chen, L.F., Shigesada, K., Murakami, Y. and Ito, Y. (1999) A WW domain-containing Yes-associated protein (YAP) is a novel transcriptional co-activator. EMBO J. **18**, 2551–2562

32. Schumacher, B., Skwarczynska, M., Rose, R. and Ottmann, C. (2010) Structure of a 14-3-3σ-YAP phosphopeptide complex at 1.15 Å resolution. Acta Crystallogr. Sect. F Struct. Biol. Crystal. Commun. **66**, 978–984

33. Salah, Z. and Aqeilan, R.I. (2011) WW domain interactions regulate the Hippo tumor suppressor pathway. Cell Death Dis. **2**, e172

34. Koepf, E.K., Petrassi, H.M., Ratnaswamy, G., Huff, M.E., Sudol, M. and Kelly, J.W. (1999) Characterization of the structure and function of W-to-F WW domain variants: identification of a natively unfolded protein that folds upon ligand binding. Biochemistry **38**, 14338–14351

35. Salah, Z., Melino, G. and Aqeilan, R.I. (2011) Negative regulation of the Hippo pathway by E3 ubiquitin ligase ITCH is sufficient to promote tumorigenicity. Cancer Res. **71**, 2010–2020

36. Ohnishi, S., Guntert, P., Koshiba, S., Tomizawa, T., Akasaka, R., Tochio, N., Sato, M., Inoue, M., Harada, T., Watanabe, S. et al. (2007) Solution structure of an atypical WW domain in a novel β-clam-like dimeric form. FEBS Lett. **581**, 462–468

37. Webb, C., Upadhyay, A., Giuntini, F., Eggleston, I., Furutani-Seiki, M., Ishima, R. and Bagby, S. (2011) Structural features and ligand binding properties of tandem WW domains from YAP and TAZ, nuclear effectors of the Hippo pathway. Biochemistry **50**, 3300–3309

38. Hwang, E., Ryu, K.S., Paakkonen, K., Guntert, P., Cheong, H.K., Lim, D.S., Lee, J.O., Jeon, Y.H. and Cheong, C. (2007) Structural insight into dimeric interaction of the SARAH domains from Mst1 and RASSF family proteins in the apoptosis pathway. Proc. Natl. Acad. Sci. U.S.A. **104**, 9236–9241

39. Hergovich, A. (2011) MOB control: reviewing a conserved family of kinase regulators. Cell. Signalling **23**, 1433–1440

40. Mrkobrada, S., Boucher, L., Ceccarelli, D.F., Tyers, M. and Sicheri, F. (2006) Structural and functional analysis of *Saccharomyces cerevisiae* Mob1. J. Mol. Biol. **362**, 430–440

41. Lee, H.J. and Zheng, J.J. (2010) PDZ domains and their binding partners: structure, specificity, and modification. Cell Commun. Signal. **8**, 8

42. Remue, E., Meerschaert, K., Oka, T., Boucherie, C., Vandekerckhove, J., Sudol, M. and Gettemans, J. (2010) TAZ interacts with zonula occludens-1 and -2 proteins in a PDZ-1 dependent manner. FEBS Lett. **584**, 4175–4180

43. Oka, T., Remue, E., Meerschaert, K., Vanloo, B., Boucherie, C., Gfeller, D., Bader, G.D., Sidhu, S.S., Vandekerckhove, J., Gettemans, J. and Sudol, M. (2010) Functional complexes between YAP2 and ZO-2 are PDZ domain-dependent, and regulate YAP2 nuclear localization and signalling. Biochem. J. **432**, 461–472

44. Alarcón, C., Zaromytidou, A.I., Xi, Q.R., Gao, S., Yu, J.Z., Fujisawa, S., Barlas, A., Miller, A.N., Manova-Todorova, K., Macias, M.J. et al. (2009) Nuclear CDKs drive Smad transcriptional activation and turnover in BMP and TGFβ pathways. Cell **139**, 757–769

45. Karpowicz, P., Perez, J. and Perrimon, N. (2010) The Hippo tumor suppressor pathway regulates intestinal stem cell regeneration. Development **137**, 4135–4145

46. Reddy, B.V.V.G., Rauskolb, C. and Irvine, K.D. (2010) Influence of Fat-Hippo and Notch signaling on the proliferation and differentiation of *Drosophila* optic neuroepithelia. Development **137**, 2397–2408

47. Fernandez, A., Northcott, P.A., Dalton, J., Fraga, C., Ellison, D., Angers, S., Taylor, M.D. and Kenney, A.M. (2009) YAP1 is amplified and up-regulated in hedgehog-associated medulloblastomas and mediates Sonic hedgehog-driven neural precursor proliferation. Genes Dev. **23**, 2729–2741

48. Choi, J., Oh, S., Lee D., Oh, H.J., Park, J.Y., Lee, S.B. and Lim, D.S. (2009) Mst1-FoxO signaling protects naïve T lymphocytes from cellular oxidative stress in mice. PloS ONE 4, e8011

49. Yuan, Z., Kim, D., Shu, S., Wu, J., Guo, J., Xiao, L., Kaneko, S., Coppola, D. and Cheng, J.Q. (2010) Phosphoinositide 3-kinase/Akt inhibits MST1-mediated pro-apoptotic signaling through phosphorylation of threonine 120. J. Biol. Chem. **285**, 3815–3824

50. Nicolay, B.N., Bayarmagnai, B., Islam, A., Lopez-Bigas, N. and Frolov, M.V. (2011) Cooperation between dE2F1 and Yki/Sd defines a distinct transcriptional program necessary to bypass cell cycle exit. Genes Dev. **25**, 323–335

51. Tschöp, K., Conery, A.R., Litovchick, L., Decaprio, J.A., Settleman, J., Harlow, E. and Dyson, N. (2011) A kinase shRNA screen links LATS2 and the pRB tumor suppressor. Genes Dev. **25**, 814–830

52. Zhang, J.M., Ji, J.Y., Yu, M., Overholtzer, M., Smolen, G.A., Wang, R., Brugge, J.S., Dyson, N.J. and Haber, D.A. (2009) YAP-dependent induction of amphiregulin identifies a non-cell-autonomous component of the Hippo pathway. Nature Cell Biol. **11**, 1444–1450

53. Kanai, F., Marignani, P.A., Sarbassova, D., Yagi, R., Hall, R.A., Donowitz, M., Hisaminato, A., Fujiwara, T., Ito, Y., Cantley, L.C. and Yaffe, M.B. (2000) TAZ: a novel transcriptional co-activator regulated by interactions with 14-3-3 and PDZ domain proteins. EMBO J. **19**, 6778–6791

54. Basu, S., Totty, N.F., Irwin, M.S., Sudol, M. and Downward, J. (2003) Akt phosphorylates the Yes-associated protein, YAP, to induce interaction with 14-3-3 and attenuation of p73-mediated apoptosis. Mol. Cell **11**, 11–23

55. Chan, S.W., Lim, C.J., Chong, Y.F., Pobbati, A.V., Huang, C.X. and Hong, W.J. (2011) Hippo pathway-independent restriction of TAZ and YAP by angiomotin. J. Biol. Chem. **286**, 7018–7026

56. Espanel, X. and Sudol, M. (2001) Yes-associated protein and p53-binding protein-2 interact through their WW and SH3 domains. J. Biol. Chem. **276**, 14514–14523

57. Sudol, M., Bork, P., Einbond, A., Kastury, K., Druck, T., Negrini, M., Huebner, K. and Lehman, D. (1995) Characterization of the mammalian Yap (Yes-associated protein) gene and its role in defining a novel protein module, the WW domain. J. Biol. Chem. **270**, 14733–14741

58. Komuro, A., Nagai, M., Navin, N.E. and Sudol, M. (2003) WW domain-containing protein YAP associates with ErbB-4 and acts as a co-transcriptional activator for the carboxyl-terminal fragment of ErbB-4 that translocates to the nucleus. J. Biol. Chem. **278**, 33334–33341

59. Badouel, C., Gardano, L., Amin, N., Garg, A., Rosenfeld, R., Le Bihan, T. and McNeill, H. (2009) The FERM-domain protein Expanded regulates Hippo pathway activity via direct interactions with the transcriptional activator Yorkie. Dev. Cell **16**, 411–420

60. Howell, M., Borchers, C. and Milgram, S.L. (2004) Heterogeneous nuclear ribonuclear protein U associates with YAP and regulates its co-activation of Bax transcription. J. Biol. Chem. **279**, 26300–26306

61. Lei, Q.Y., Zhang, H., Zhao, B., Zha, Z.Y., Bai, F., Pei, X.H., Zhao, S., Xiong, Y. and Guan, K.L. (2008) TAZ promotes cell proliferation and epithelial-mesenchymal transition and is inhibited by the Hippo pathway. Mol. Cell. Biol. **28**, 2426–2436

62. Zhang, J., Smolen, G.A. and Haber, D.A. (2008) Negative regulation of YAP by LATS1 underscores evolutionary conservation of the *Drosophila* Hippo pathway. Cancer Res. **68**, 2789–2794

63. Gavva, N.R., Gavva, R., Ermekova, K., Sudol, M. and Shen, C.K.J. (1997) Interaction of WW domains with hematopoietic transcription factor p45/NF-E2 and RNA polymerase II. J. Biol. Chem. **272**, 24105–24108

64. Mohler, P.J., Kreda, S.M., Boucher, R.C., Sudol, M., Stutts, M.J. and Milgram, S.L. (1999) Yes-associated protein 65 localizes p62 (c-Yes) to the apical compartment of airway epithelia by association with EBP50. J. Cell Biol. **147**, 879–890

65. Strano, S., Monti, O., Baccarini, A., Sudol, M., Sacchi, A. and Blandino, G. (2001) Physical interaction with yes-associated protein enhances p73 transcriptional activity. Eur. J. Cancer **37**, S279

66. Oka, T. and Sudol, M. (2009) Nuclear localization and pro-apoptotic signaling of YAP2 require intact PDZ-binding motif. Genes Cells **14**, 607–615

67. Hong, J.H., Hwang, E.S., McManus, M.T., Amsterdam, A., Tian, Y., Kalmukova, R., Mueller, E., Benjamin, T., Spiegelman, B.M., Sharp, P.A. et al. (2005) TAZ, a transcriptional modulator of mesenchymal stem cell differentiation. Science **309**, 1074–1078

68. Kulman, J.D., Harris, J.E., Xie, L. and Davie, E.W. (2007) Proline-rich Gla protein 2 is a cell-surface vitamin K-dependent protein that binds to the transcriptional coactivator Yes-associated protein. Proc. Natl. Acad. Sci. U.S.A. **104**, 8767–8772

69. Zaidi, S.K., Sullivan, A.J., Medina, R., Ito, Y., van Wijnen, A.J., Stein, J.L., Lian, J.B. and Stein, G.S. (2004) Tyrosine phosphorylation controls Runx2-mediated subnuclear targeting of YAP to repress transcription. EMBO J. **23**, 790–799

70. Vassilev, A., Kaneko, K.J., Shu, H.J., Zhao, Y.M. and DePamphilis, M.L. (2001) TEAD/TEF transcription factors utilize the activation domain of YAP65, a Src/Yes-associated protein localized in the cytoplasm. Genes Dev. **15**, 1229–1241

71. Chen, H.I. and Sudol, M. (1995) The WW domain of Yes-associated protein binds a proline-rich ligand that differs from the consensus established for Src homology 3-binding modules. Proc. Natl. Acad. Sci. U.S.A. **92**, 7819–7823

© The Authors Journal compilation © 2012 Biochemical Society
Essays Biochem. (2012) 53, 129–140: doi: 10.1042/BSE0530129

10

Epithelial cell polarity: what flies can teach us about cancer

Daniel T. Bergstralh and Daniel St Johnston[1]

The Gurdon Institute and the Department of Genetics, University of Cambridge, Tennis Court Road, Cambridge CB2 1QN, U.K.

Abstract

Epithelial cells are polarized along their apical–basal axis. Much of the cellular machinery that goes into establishing and maintaining epithelial cell polarity is evolutionarily conserved. Model organisms, including the fruit fly, *Drosophila melanogaster*, are thus particularly useful for the study of cell polarity. Work in *Drosophila* has identified several important components of the polarity machinery and has also established the surprising existence of a secondary cell polarity pathway required only under conditions of energetic stress. This work has important implications for the understanding of human cancer. Most cancers are epithelial in origin, and the loss of cell polarity is a critical step towards malignancy. Thus a better understanding of how polarity is established and maintained in epithelial cells will help us to understand the process of malignant transformation and may lead to improved therapies. In the present chapter we discuss the current understanding of how epithelial cell polarity is regulated and the known associations between polarity factors and cancer.

[1]*To whom correspondence should be addressed (email d.stjohnston@gurdon. cam.ac.uk).*

Introduction

Multicellularity requires the organization of cells into specialized tissues. The cells that make up epithelial tissue are polarized along their apicobasal axes, and this polarity is crucial to their function, which may be absorptive (as in the gut), secretory (as in the glands) or protective (as in the skin). In epithelial cells polarity is driven by mutually exclusive apical, lateral and basal cortical regions. These regions are defined in large part by two cell–cell junctions which act to separate them: the AJ (adherens junction), which joins cells together in an epithelial sheet, and the septate junction (in insects) or TJ (tight junction) (in vertebrates), which acts as a barrier to paracellular diffusion (Figure 1). Notably, the arrangement of these junctions typically differs between insect and vertebrate cells. In the former, the AJ usually localizes apically to (above) the septate junction. In vertebrates, the opposite is true (Figure 1).

Despite this key difference, the regulation of epithelial polarity is substantially conserved between flies and humans. In fact, much of our understanding of epithelial polarity derives from studies in *Drosophila*. This model system has a number of advantages over cell-culture-based work. Flies can be easily dissected for convincing imaging of cells within the context of a tissue. They are also genetically tractable, so that polarity factors may be identified and manipulated. Work in flies, *Caenorhabditis elegans* and other systems has defined a number of signalling modules acting at each cortical region to establish and maintain epithelial polarity. Recent work in *Drosophila* has also revealed the

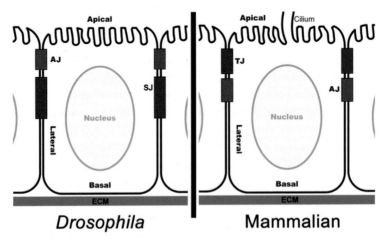

Figure 1. Cell polarity in *Drosophila* and mammalian epithelial cells
Three cortical regions are defined; apical (shown here at the top, with microvilli), lateral (facing adjacent cells) and basal (facing a basement membrane). Cell polarity is substantially defined by two cell–cell junctions, the AJ and either the septate junction (SJ) or the TJ. In insect cells the AJ is typically apical to the septate junction. In mammalian cells it is basal to the TJ.

surprising finding that regulation of polarity requires an additional signalling pathway under conditions of cellular energy deprivation.

The factors that control epithelial polarity are under increasing scrutiny for their association with cancer. Approximately 80–90% of all human tumours are epithelial in origin [1]. The progression of cancer to malignancy and metastasis is marked by the EMT (epithelial–mesenchymal transition), a change in cell architecture and behaviour characterized in large part by the loss of cell polarity. The loss or misregulation of cell polarity factors may then be a key event in tumour progression. Investigation of the low-energy polarity pathway is likely to prove particularly important for understanding malignancy, as tumour progression characteristically includes a period in which cancerous cells are deprived of energy. In the present chapter we review the factors that regulate polarity in both normal and low-energy conditions, and what has been learned so far about the relationship of these factors to cancer.

Apical signalling factors

The Crb (Crumbs) complex

The Crb complex is comprised of three key components, Crb, Sdt (Stardust) and PATJ [PALS1 (protein associated with lin seven 1)-associated TJ protein], as well as the less well-defined components Lin7, Moesin, Yurt and β_H-Spectrin (Figure 2) [2]. Crb is critical to establishment of the apical domain. The loss of Crb function prevents formation of the apical domain entirely, whereas Crb overexpression results in an expansion of the apical domain and corresponding loss of the lateral domain (reviewed in [3]). Recent work from the Laprise laboratory demonstrates that this effect relies on a balance of signalling between Crb and a signalling module consisting of PI3K (phosphoinositide 3-kinase) and the Rho-family GTPase Rac1 [4].

A mammalian orthologue of Crb, called Crb3, appears to play an analogous role to *Drosophila* Crb in the establishment and maintenance of epithelial cell polarity. Overexpression of Crb3 promotes expansion of the apical domain in vertebrate cells [5]. An additional function of Crb3 in vertebrate cells is the organization of TJs [6,7].

Crb3 is implicated in tumour development and metastasis. A study by Karp et al. [8] demonstrated that immortalized murine epithelial cells selected for tumorigenicity when transplanted into mice lost expression of Crb. This loss was associated with phenotypic changes characteristic of EMT: disrupted polarity, failure to form TJs, and the loss of contact inhibition *in vitro*. Retrovirus-mediated re-introduction of Crb3 rescued these features and prevented metastasis [8]. Although these findings suggest that Crb3 protects cells from transformation by ensuring that cell polarity is maintained, it is important to note that the tumour suppressive function of Crb3 might be attributed only in part to its role in regulating polarity. Work in *Drosophila* has demonstrated that

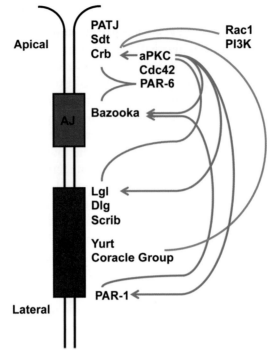

Figure 2. A visual overview of epithelial cell polarity complexes in *Drosophila*, their positions in the cell, and some known interactions between them
Phosphorylation is indicated by green arrows and direct binding is indicated by orange. Interactions of an unknown or potentially indirect nature are shown in blue. PATJ, PALSI-associated TJ protein; PI3K, phosphoinositide 3-kinase; SJ, septate junction.

Crb is a regulator of the Hippo-Yorkie pathway, which controls tissue size and is also implicated in cancer development [9,10].

aPKC (atypical protein kinase C), Cdc42 (cell division cycle 42) and PAR (PARtitioning defective)-6

Three additional factors, aPKC, Cdc42 and the scaffolding protein PAR-6, also act at the apical cortex to regulate epithelial polarity (Figure 2). Although earlier work suggested that these proteins participate in a complex with the polarity factor Bazooka (PAR-3 in mammals), this view is being refined. Increasing evidence derived from flies and mammalian cells indicates that they work together with Crb to regulate Bazooka and other factors both through phosphorylation and by physical association (reviewed in [3]). Crb itself is a substrate for aPKC and this phosphorylation is required for apical localization of the Crb complex [11].

Accumulated evidence links these proteins to cancer. In flies, the expression of constitutively active aPKC causes epithelial disorganization and overgrowth, suggestive of tumorigenesis [11,12]. aPKCı, one of two human orthologues of *Drosophila* aPKC, is frequently amplified and overexpressed in colon carcinomas and non-small-cell lung cancers, suggesting that overactive aPKC contributes to carcinogenesis in humans, as it does in flies [13–15]. More classical oncogenes can also function, at least in part, by disrupting the regulation of the PAR-6–aPKC complex. Activated ErbB2 associates with PAR-6–aPKC to promote the loss of epithelial architecture and reduced apoptosis in an *in vitro* model for breast cancer [16]. Furthermore, PAR-6 acts downstream of TGFβ (transforming growth factor β) receptors and in partnership with the ubiquitin ligase Smurf to induce degradation of the cytoskeleton regulator RhoA, thus in turn promoting EMT [17].

Bazooka

Bazooka is required to position the AJ, which separates the lateral from the apical domain (Figure 2) [2]. The positioning of Bazooka requires an intricate system of regulation. Bazooka appears to cycle between a state in which it is bound to PAR-6 and a state in which it is not [18]. Recent work has demonstrated that disassociation is promoted by two events [18]. The first is competition with Crb, which can bind PAR-6 and prevent interaction with Bazooka. The second is phosphorylation of Bazooka by aPKC, which weakens the interaction between Bazooka and PAR-6. [18]. Similarly, during cell polarization in the developing *Drosophila* embryo, phosphorylation of Bazooka by aPKC weakens a transient association of Bazooka with Sdt, allowing for the Crb complex to form [19].

The mammalian orthologue of Bazooka is PAR-3. It appears to have a similar role in organizing polarity, although with an important difference. Whereas Bazooka is required for generating the AJ in flies, PAR-3 is required for the formation of TJs in mammals [20]. As discussed earlier, these two types of junction have different functions, but their positions within the cell are similar (Figure 1). Thus it seems that Bazooka and PAR-3 are required to position the most apical junctional complex, regardless of its function.

A potential role for PAR-3 in human cancer has been addressed only recently. Two studies have shown that PAR-3 is down-regulated or mutated in a number of human carcinomas and cell lines [21,22]. The rescue of PAR-3 function in two such cell lines both re-established TJs and slowed cell growth [22]. Thus PAR-3 appears to be acting as a tumour suppressive factor.

Basolateral signalling factors

PAR-1

Basal to the AJ, along the basolateral cortex, a number of pathways act in opposition to the apical signalling complexes in defining polarity. The kinase PAR-1 regulates Bazooka by targeting it directly, consequently preventing the AJ from expanding basally along the lateral cortex (Figure 2) [23]. As with the Crb complex, regulation of PAR-1 by aPKC is also important. In mammalian cells, phosphorylation of PAR-1 by aPKC is required for PAR-1 localization and activity [24]. The regulation of PAR-1 during tumour development has not yet been studied.

The Scribble complex

Lgl (lethal giant larvae), Dlg (Discs large) and Scrib (Scribble) make up the Scribble complex of proteins, another important basolateral polarity pathway (Figure 2) [25]. These proteins are required for formation of the septate junction (reviewed in [3]). As with PAR-1, Scribble complex proteins act to oppose apical polarity signalling. Lgl binds to the PAR-6–aPKC complex to inhibit its activity and cortical association, whereas aPKC phosphorylation of Lgl excludes the latter from the apical cortex [26,27].

Of the normal energy signalling complexes, the Scribble complex has potentially the clearest association with tumorigenic phenotypes in the fly. *lgl*, *dlg* and *scrib* are nTSGs (neoplastic tumour suppressor genes); loss-of-function in any of these proteins promotes both the loss of cell polarity and concomitant overproliferation, resulting in a phenotype reminiscent of human tumorigenesis. [25]. When combined with overactive oncogenes, such as Ras, these tumours can become metastatic [28,29]. Likewise, the loss of human Scribble promotes an invasive phenotype in cells with overactive Ras [30].

The story is likely to be more complex in humans than in flies, as mammals have multiple orthologues of each Scribble complex member [3]. However, the relevance of these factors to human cancer is underlined by a number of recent studies in mammalian systems. Decreased expression of the human orthologue of Lgl, Hugl-1, has been observed in multiple cancer types, with the degree of loss correlating with disease progression and metastasis [31–33]. Likewise, human Scribble is commonly deregulated in mammary carcinomas, either at the level of expression or localization [34]. Furthermore, both Scribble and Dlg-1 are known targets for viral oncoproteins, which may bind these proteins and disrupt their function (reviewed in [35]).

Yurt and the Coracle group

A second set of septate junction proteins, composed of Yurt and the Coracle group proteins Cora (Coracle), Neurexin IV and Na$^+$/K$^+$-ATPase is also involved in regulating epithelial cell polarity in *Drosophila* (Figure 2). Yurt appears to function in parallel with a module comprising the other three proteins, which, unlike Yurt, are required for septate junction formation [36,37]. Interestingly these proteins are required for polarity only during the organogenesis stage of embryo development, during which they act to oppose Crb signalling. In embryos doubly mutant for Yurt and a Coracle group protein, apical boundaries are stretched, as they are upon Crb overexpression [37]. When Crb function is lost, mutation of Yurt and any one of the Coracle group genes rescues polarity [37].

The mammalian Lulu proteins (Lulu1/2) are candidate orthologues of Yurt. Recent work has demonstrated that these proteins localize basolaterally in epithelial cells, where they act to regulate cell shape [38]. The expression and regulation of these proteins in cancer has not yet been examined.

The low-energy polarity pathway

LKB1 (liver kinase B1) and AMPK (AMP-activated kinase)

LKB1 and its target AMPK comprise a signalling module responsible for sensing low cellular energy, as indicated by a high concentration of cellular AMP, and act to inhibit processes that use up ATP and to activate processes that generate ATP. Under low-energy conditions, disruption of either AMPK or LKB1 function yields strong cell polarity defects in the follicle cell epithelium, a single layer of epithelial tissue that surrounds the developing oocyte [39]. These defects are rescued by the expression of a constitutively active phospho-mimetic AMPKα in *lkb1* mutants [39]. Importantly, maintenance of cell polarity under normal-energy conditions is AMPK-independent; *ampk* mutant cells only exhibit epithelial polarity defects under starvation [39].

Cell polarity defects are also observed in *ampk* or *lkb1* mutant *Drosophila* embryos, suggesting that at this stage of development the fly may be under low-energy conditions [40]. In embryos, the myosin regulatory light chain [called Sqh (spaghetti-squash) in flies] is an important downstream mediator of LKB1-AMPK polarity signalling (Figure 3) [40]. Conservation of this pathway in human cells has already been established; low-energy polarity signalling through LKB1-AMPK has been demonstrated in the human colon carcinoma cell line LS174T [40].

With regard to cancer, low-energy polarity is particularly worthy of attention. It has long been recognized that malignant cells derive their cellular energy from a much higher rate of glycolysis (a characteristic known as the Warburg effect) than do healthy cells. The transition to a high glycolytic state as tumour cells become malignant is probably initiated to compensate for a loss of available oxygen within the growing tumour and resultant depleted energy stores in the cell. At this transition point the low-energy polarity pathway may act as a crucial check against further transformation. The loss of this pathway would thus open the door to malignancy.

LKB1-AMPK signalling is specifically implicated in the suppression of epithelium-derived cancers. LKB1 is a well-known tumour suppressor in epithelial tissues. Mutation of *LKB1* is associated with Peutz–Jeghers syndrome, a condition characterized by increased risk of epithelial cancers and gastrointestinal polyps, and *LKB1* is also commonly mutated in non-small-cell lung cancers and cervical cancers [41,42]. The tumour suppressor function of LKB1 is thought to be mediated through AMPK [43].

Evidence connecting AMPK with cancer is provided by epidemiological studies of patients with T2DM (Type 2 diabetes mellitus). These patients are commonly treated with the drug metformin, which decreases available energy in the cell by acting as a mitochondrial poison. While T2DM patients demonstrate a significantly increased cancer risk, long-term treatment with metformin is associated with a decreased risk of cancer in an approximately dose-dependent

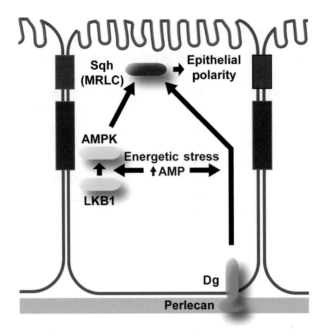

Figure 3. Recent work in *Drosophila* and the mammalian colon carcinoma cell line LS174T has revealed a second signalling pathway that controls cell polarity under conditions of energetic stress

LKB1/AMPK is activated in response to a high AMP/ATP ratio, leading to the activation of Sqh and the maintenance of polarity. Dg, in partnership with its extracellular ligand perlecan, is also required for low-energy cell polarity. These factors are required for the phosphorylation of Sqh, but also for its intracellular localization, which is apical under low-energy conditions. MRLC, myosin regulatory light chain.

manner [44]. Both the anti-cancer and anti-diabetic effects of metformin are mediated by AMPK [45].

Importantly, the cancer-limiting effect of AMPK stimulation is not restricted to T2DM patients. Metformin acts to inhibit the proliferation of breast cancer cells *in vitro* [46], and metformin and other AMPK-stimulating agents delay tumour onset in cancer prone *Pten*^+/− mice (PTEN is phosphatase and tensin homologue deleted on chromosome 10) [47]. In contrast, inhibition of AMPK accelerates tumorigenesis in these same mice [47]. Several studies have also demonstrated decreased cancer incidence in mice fed a calorie-restricted diet. Cumulatively, these findings suggest the possibility that low-energy-induced AMPK signalling helps to protect cells from transformation by ensuring that polarity is maintained.

Dg (dystroglycan)

Located at the basal cortex, Dg is one of several receptors that interact with components of the ECM (extracellular matrix). Under normal energy conditions, neither Dg nor its ECM ligand perlecan are required to maintain epithelial polarity, but both factors are required for polarity under energetic stress (Figure 3) [48]. The relationship between these factors and the rest of the low-energy polarity pathway is complex. Although Dg is required for the phosphorylation of Sqh, this activity is independent of AMPK. Furthermore, the expression of phospho-mimetic Sqh is not sufficient to rescue the polarity phenotype of Dg-mutant cells. Instead Dg may be necessary to regulate the intracellular localization of Sqh. In starved cells Sqh localizes apically in the presence of Dg, but basally in its absence.

Dg is also implicated in cancer. Its expression is frequently decreased in a variety of tumour types, indicating that its function is lost during cell transformation [49]. Furthermore, exogenous overexpression of Dg inhibits the tumorigenicity of transformed human breast epithelial cells [50]. This evidence suggests that Dg acts as a protective factor against cancer, perhaps through its role in regulating low-energy polarity.

Conclusion

The establishment and maintenance of epithelial cell polarity presents a rich and intricate problem for study, and the fruit fly has proved an outstanding tool. Polarity factors, of which many are known already, continue to be identified in *Drosophila* and other organisms. Current work is focused on deciphering the complex molecular relationships between these factors and between the pathways in which they participate. These pathways can appear to act in opposition, redundantly, in a tissue-specific manner, or most intriguingly, in a manner dependent on the energy status of the cell.

The connection between cancer and polarity regulation is evidently important, but only beginning to be researched in depth. Malignant transformation is marked by the loss of cell polarity, and as discussed above, several polarity factors are known to be lost or mutated in certain tumours. To date these findings are largely correlative and merit further exploration. The regulation of polarity under low-energy conditions deserves particular scrutiny, as links between energy status and cancer are well established at the level of both the organism and the cell. Several important questions surround the low-energy polarity pathway: (i) how is Sqh, which makes up part of an actin motor protein, involved in regulating polarity? (ii) How does the ECM receptor Dg, which is required independently of AMPK for the phosphorylation of Sqh, relate to other members of the pathway? (iii) What additional factors are involved?

As the answers to these questions emerge we are likely to have an improved understanding of malignant transformation and how to address it. Therapeutic strategies aimed towards protecting epithelial cell polarity may prove useful in the treatment and prevention of cancer, and we will continue to owe the fruit fly for its important role in illuminating human biology and disease.

Summary

- *The machinery that controls the establishment and maintenance of epithelial cell polarity is largely conserved among animals.*
- *Drosophila is thus a useful model system for the study of polarity regulation, and much of our understanding of polarity is derived from work in flies and other model organisms.*
- *A number of polarity pathways act at different regions of the cell cortex, often in opposition with one another.*
- *The loss of epithelial cell polarity is a hallmark event of malignant transformation.*
- *Several polarity factors have been shown to be lost or misregulated in diverse tumour types.*
- *Under energetic stress, signalling mediated by LKB1, AMPK, Dg and Sqh (myosin regulatory light chain) is required for the maintenance of epithelial cell polarity.*
- *Multiple lines of evidence connect low-energy states with cancer, suggesting that low-energy polarity signalling may be of particular importance to tumorigenesis.*

References

1. Molitoris, B.A. and Nelson, W.J. (1990) Alterations in the establishment and maintenance of epithelial cell polarity as a basis for disease processes. J. Clin. Invest. **85**, 3–9
2. Laprise, P. and Tepass, U. (2011) Novel insights into epithelial polarity proteins in *Drosophila*. Trends Cell Biol. **21**, 401–408
3. St Johnston, D. and Ahringer, J. (2010) Cell polarity in eggs and epithelia: parallels and diversity. Cell **141**, 757–774
4. Chartier, F.J.-M., Hardy, E.J.-L. and Laprise, P. (2011) Crumbs controls epithelial integrity by inhibiting Rac1 and PI3K. J. Cell Sci. **124**, 3393–3398
5. Chalmers, A.D. (2005) aPKC, Crumbs3 and Lgl2 control apicobasal polarity in early vertebrate development Development **132**, 977–986
6. Lemmers, C., Michel, D., Lane-Guermonprez, L., Delgrossi, M.-H., Médina, E., Arsanto, J.-P. and Le Bivic, A. (2004) CRB3 binds directly to Par6 and regulates the morphogenesis of the tight junctions in mammalian epithelial cells. Mol. Biol. Cell **15**, 1324–1333
7. Fogg, V.C., Liu, C.-J. and Margolis, B. (2005) Multiple regions of Crumbs3 are required for tight junction formation in MCF10A cells. J. Cell Sci. **118**, 2859–2869
8. Karp, C.M., Tan, T.T., Mathew, R., Nelson, D., Mukherjee, C., Degenhardt, K., Karantza-Wadsworth, V. and White, E. (2008) Role of the polarity determinant crumbs in suppressing mammalian epithelial tumor progression. Cancer Res. **68**, 4105–4115
9. Chen, C.-L., Gajewski, K.M., Hamaratoglu, F., Bossuyt, W., Sansores-Garcia, L., Tao, C. and Halder, G. (2010) The apical-basal cell polarity determinant Crumbs regulates Hippo signaling in *Drosophila*. Proc. Natl. Acad. Sci. U.S.A. **107**, 15810–15815
10. Ling, C., Zheng, Y., Yin, F., Yu, J., Huang, J., Hong, Y., Wu, S. and Pan, D. (2010) The apical transmembrane protein Crumbs functions as a tumor suppressor that regulates Hippo signaling by binding to Expanded. Proc. Natl. Acad. Sci. U.S.A. **107**, 10532–10537
11. Sotillos, S., Díaz-Meco, M.T., Caminero, E., Moscat, J. and Campuzano, S. (2004) DaPKC-dependent phosphorylation of Crumbs is required for epithelial cell polarity in *Drosophila*. J. Cell Biol. **166**, 549–557

12. Grifoni, D., Garoia, F., Bellosta, P., Parisi, F., De Biase, D., Collina, G., Strand, D., Cavicchi, S. and Pession, A. (2007) aPKCζ cortical loading is associated with Lgl cytoplasmic release and tumor growth in *Drosophila* and human epithelia. Oncogene **26**, 5960–5965

13. Murray, N.R., Jamieson, L., Yu, W., Zhang, J., Gökmen-Polar, Y., Sier, D., Anastasiadis, P., Gatalica, Z., Thompson, E.A. and Fields, A.P. (2004) Protein kinase Cι is required for Ras transformation and colon carcinogenesis *in vivo*. J. Cell Biol. **164**, 797–802

14. Regala, R., Weems, C. and Jamieson, L. (2005) Atypical protein kinase Cι plays a critical role in human lung cancer cell growth and tumorigenicity J. Biol. Chem. **280**, 31109–31115

15. Regala, R., Weems, C., Jamieson, L. and Khoor, A. (2005) Atypical protein kinase Cι is an oncogene in human non-small cell lung cancer. Cancer Res. **65**, 8905–8911

16. Aranda, V., Haire, T., Nolan, M.E., Calarco, J.P., Rosenberg, A.Z., Fawcett, J.P., Pawson, T. and Muthuswamy, S.K. (2006) Par6-aPKC uncouples ErbB2 induced disruption of polarized epithelial organization from proliferation control. Nat. Cell Biol. **8**, 1235–1245

17. Ozdamar, B., Bose, R., Barrios-Rodiles, M., Wang, H.-R., Zhang, Y. and Wrana, J.L. (2005) Regulation of the polarity protein Par6 by TGFβ receptors controls epithelial cell plasticity. Science **307**, 1603–1609

18. Morais-de-Sá, E., Mirouse, V. and St Johnston, D. (2010) aPKC phosphorylation of Bazooka defines the apical/lateral border in *Drosophila* epithelial cells. Cell **141**, 509–523

19. Krahn, M.P., Buckers, J., Kastrup, L. and Wodarz, A. (2010) Formation of a Bazooka-Stardust complex is essential for plasma membrane polarity in epithelia. J. Cell Biol. **190**, 751–760

20. Chen, X. and Macara, I.G. (2005) Par-3 controls tight junction assembly through the Rac exchange factor Tiam1. Nat. Cell Biol. **7**, 262–269

21. Zen, K., Yasui, K., Gen, Y., Dohi, O., Wakabayashi, N., Mitsufuji, S., Itoh, Y., Zen, Y., Nakanuma, Y., Taniwaki, M. et al. (2009) Defective expression of polarity protein PAR-3 gene (PARD3) in esophageal squamous cell carcinoma. Oncogene **28**, 2910–2918

22. Rothenberg, S.M., Mohapatra, G., Rivera, M.N., Winokur, D., Greninger, P., Nitta, M., Sadow, P.M., Sooriyakumar, G., Brannigan, B.W., Ulman, M.J. et al. (2010) A genome-wide screen for microdeletions reveals disruption of polarity complex genes in diverse human cancers. Cancer Res. **70**, 2158–2164

23. Benton, R. and St Johnston, D. (2003) *Drosophila* PAR-1 and 14-3-3 inhibit Bazooka/PAR-3 to establish complementary cortical domains in polarized cells. Cell **115**, 691–704

24. Hurov, J.B., Watkins, J.L. and Piwnica-Worms, H. (2004) Atypical PKC phosphorylates PAR-1 kinases to regulate localization and activity. Curr. Biol. **14**, 736–741

25. Bilder, D. (2004) Epithelial polarity and proliferation control: links from the *Drosophila* neoplastic tumor suppressors. Genes Dev. **18**, 1909–1925

26. Betschinger, J., Mechtler, K. and Knoblich, J.A. (2003) The Par complex directs asymmetric cell division by phosphorylating the cytoskeletal protein Lgl. Nature **422**, 326–330

27. Hutterer, A., Betschinger, J., Petronczki, M. and Knoblich, J.A. (2004) Sequential roles of Cdc42, Par-6, aPKC, and Lgl in the establishment of epithelial polarity during *Drosophila* embryogenesis. Dev. Cell **6**, 845–854

28. Brumby, A.M. and Richardson, H.E. (2003) Scribble mutants cooperate with oncogenic Ras or Notch to cause neoplastic overgrowth in *Drosophila*. EMBO J. **22**, 5769–5779

29. Pagliarini, R.A. and Xu, T. (2003) A genetic screen in *Drosophila* for metastatic behavior. Science **302**, 1227–1231

30. Dow, L.E., Elsum, I.A., King, C.L., Kinross, K.M., Richardson, H.E. and Humbert, P.O. (2008) Loss of human Scribble cooperates with H-Ras to promote cell invasion through deregulation of MAPK signalling. Oncogene **27**, 5988–6001

31. Schimanski, C.C., Schmitz, G., Kashyap, A., Bosserhoff, A.K., Bataille, F., Schäfer, S.C., Lehr, H.A., Berger, M.R., Galle, P.R., Strand, S. and Strand, D. (2005) Reduced expression of Hugl-1, the human homologue of *Drosophila* tumour suppressor gene lgl, contributes to progression of colorectal cancer. Oncogene **24**, 3100–3109

32. Kuphal, S., Wallner, S., Schimanski, C.C., Bataille, F., Hofer, P., Strand, S., Strand, D. and Bosserhoff, A.K. (2006) Expression of Hugl-1 is strongly reduced in malignant melanoma. Oncogene **25**, 103–110

33. Tsuruga, T., Nakagawa, S., Watanabe, M., Takizawa, S., Matsumoto, Y., Nagasaka, K., Sone, K., Hiraike, H., Miyamoto, Y., Hiraike, O. et al. (2007) Loss of Hugl-1 expression associates with lymph node metastasis in endometrial cancer. Oncol. Res. **16**, 431–435

34. Zhan, L., Rosenberg, A., Bergami, K.C., Yu, M., Xuan, Z., Jaffe, A.B., Allred, C. and Muthuswamy, S.K. (2008) Deregulation of scribble promotes mammary tumorigenesis and reveals a role for cell polarity in carcinoma. Cell **135**, 865–878

35. Humbert, P.O., Grzeschik, N.A., Brumby, A.M., Galea, R., Elsum, I. and Richardson, H.E. (2008) Control of tumourigenesis by the Scribble/Dlg/Lgl polarity module. Oncogene **27**, 6888–6907

36. Lamb, R.S., Ward, R.E., Schweizer, L. and Fehon, R.G. (1998) *Drosophila* coracle, a member of the protein 4.1 superfamily, has essential structural functions in the septate junctions and developmental functions in embryonic and adult epithelial cells. Mol. Biol. Cell **9**, 3505–3519

37. Laprise, P., Lau, K.M., Harris, K.P., Silva-Gagliardi, N.F., Paul, S.M., Beronja, S., Beitel, G.J., McGlade, C.J. and Tepass, U. (2009) Yurt, Coracle, Neurexin IV and the Na^+, K^+-ATPase form a novel group of epithelial polarity proteins. Nature **459**, 1141–1145

38. Nakajima, H. and Tanoue, T. (2010) Epithelial cell shape is regulated by Lulu proteins via myosin-II. J. Cell Sci. **123**, 555–566

39. Mirouse, V., Swick, L.L., Kazgan, N., St Johnston, D. and Brenman, J.E. (2007) LKB1 and AMPK maintain epithelial cell polarity under energetic stress. J. Cell Biol. **177**, 387–392

40. Lee, J.H., Koh, H., Kim, M., Kim, Y., Lee, S.Y., Karess, R.E., Lee, S.-H., Shong, M., Kim, J.-M., Kim, J. and Chung, J. (2007) Energy-dependent regulation of cell structure by AMP-activated protein kinase. Nature **447**, 1017–1020

41. Hearle, N., Schumacher, V., Menko, F.H., Olschwang, S., Boardman, L.A., Gille, J.J.P., Keller, J.J., Westerman, A.M., Scott, R.J., Lim, W. et al. (2006) Frequency and spectrum of cancers in the Peutz–Jeghers syndrome. Clin. Cancer Res. **12**, 3209–3215

42. Wingo, S.N., Gallardo, T.D., Akbay, E.A., Liang, M.-C., Contreras, C.M., Boren, T., Shimamura, T., Miller, D.S., Sharpless, N.E., Bardeesy, N. et al. (2009) Somatic LKB1 mutations promote cervical cancer progression. PLoS ONE **4**, e5137

43. Kahn, B.B., Alquier, T., Carling, D. and Hardie, D.G. (2005) AMP-activated protein kinase: ancient energy gauge provides clues to modern understanding of metabolism. Cell. Metab. **1**, 15–25

44. Li, D. (2011) Metformin as an antitumor agent in cancer prevention and treatment. J. Diabetes **3**, 320–327

45. Hawley, S.A., Ross, F.A., Chevtzoff, C., Green, K.A., Evans, A., Fogarty, S., Towler, M.C., Brown, L.J., Ogunbayo, O.A., Evans, A.M. and Hardie, D.G. (2010) Use of cells expressing γ subunit variants to identify diverse mechanisms of AMPK activation. Cell. Metab. **11**, 554–565

46. Zakikhani, M., Dowling, R., Fantus, I.G., Sonenberg, N. and Pollak, M. (2006) Metformin is an AMP kinase-dependent growth inhibitor for breast cancer cells. Cancer Res. **66**, 10269–10273

47. Huang, X., Wullschleger, S., Shpiro, N., McGuire, V.A., Sakamoto, K., Woods, Y.L., McBurnie, W., Fleming, S. and Alessi, D.R. (2008) Important role of the LKB1-AMPK pathway in suppressing tumorigenesis in PTEN-deficient mice. Biochem. J. **412**, 211–221

48. Mirouse, V., Christoforou, C., Fritsch, C. and St, D. (2009) Dystroglycan and perlecan provide a basal cue required for epithelial polarity during energetic stress. Dev. Cell **16**, 83–92

49. Sgambato, A., Camerini, A., Amoroso, D., Genovese, G., De Luca, F., Cecchi, M., Migaldi, M., Rettino, A., Valsuani, C., Tartarelli, G. et al. (2007) Expression of dystroglycan correlates with tumor grade and predicts survival in renal cell carcinoma. Cancer Biol. Ther. **6**, 1840–1846

50. Sgambato, A., Camerini, A., Faraglia, B., Pavoni, E., Montanari, M., Spada, D., Losasso, C., Brancaccio, A. and Cittadini, A. (2004) Increased expression of dystroglycan inhibits the growth and tumorigenicity of human mammary epithelial cells. Cancer Biol. Ther. **3**, 967–975

© The Authors Journal compilation © 2012 Biochemical Society
Essays Biochem. (2012) **53**, 141–168: doi: 10.1042/BSE0530141

The Scribble–Dlg–Lgl polarity module in development and cancer: from flies to man

Imogen Elsum[*], Laura Yates[*], Patrick O. Humbert[*†‡§1] and Helena E. Richardson[†§‖¶]

[*]*Cell Cycle and Cancer Genetics Laboratory, Research Division, Peter MacCallum Cancer Center, Melbourne, Victoria, Australia,* [†]*Sir Peter MacCallum Department of Oncology, University of Melbourne, Melbourne 3010, Victoria, Australia,* [‡]*Department of Pathology, University of Melbourne, Melbourne 3010, Victoria, Australia,* [§]*Department of Biochemistry & Molecular Biology, University of Melbourne, Melbourne 3010, Victoria, Australia,* [‖]*Cell Cycle and Development Laboratory, Research Division, Peter MacCallum Cancer Center, Melbourne, Victoria, Australia, and* [¶]*Department of Anatomy & Cell Biology, University of Melbourne, Melbourne 3010, Victoria, Australia*

Abstract

The Scribble, Par and Crumbs modules were originally identified in the vinegar (fruit) fly, *Drosophila melanogaster*, as being critical regulators of apico–basal cell polarity. In the present chapter we focus on the Scribble polarity module, composed of Scribble, discs large and lethal giant larvae. Since the discovery of the role of the Scribble polarity module in apico–basal cell polarity, these proteins have also been recognized as having important roles in other forms of polarity,

[1]*To whom correspondence should be addressed (email Patrick.humbert@peter-mac.org).*

as well as regulation of the actin cytoskeleton, cell signalling and vesicular trafficking. In addition to these physiological roles, an important role for polarity proteins in cancer progression has also been uncovered, with loss of polarity and tissue architecture being strongly correlated with metastatic disease.

Introduction

Within a multicellular organism, cells exhibit different shapes, from the columnar epithelial cells that make up the skin and line the lung airways to the stellate fibroblast cells that make up the dermis of the skin and the migratory immune cells. Cell shape is fundamentally important during development for morphological movements and in tissue homoeostasis for cellular function and in defining tissue architecture. The deregulation of mechanisms regulating cell shape can lead to developmental disorders, tissue degeneration or cancer [1,2].

The shape of a cell depends on its cell polarity. Cell polarity can be loosely described as the asymmetric distribution of cellular constituents, including proteins, carbohydrates and lipids, to distinct cellular domains. Polarity is essential for many biological functions and plays a crucial role in processes as diverse as the growth of budding yeast, cell division, the transmission of nerve impulses, cell crawling and lymphocyte homing [3]. Several different types of cell polarity exist, including apico–basal, asymmetric cell division, planar and front–rear (migration) polarity [4–6].

ABCP (apico–basal cell polarity) defines the axis separating the apical and basal domains within a cell, and is established and maintained by the interplay between three evolutionarily conserved polarity modules, which define specialized domains along the apico–basal axis of a cell [7,8]. Establishing these cellular domains is important for the positioning of the adherens junction (composed predominantly of E-cadherin, α-catenin and β-catenin) and tight junctions [composed predominantly of ZOs (zona occludens), claudins and occludin] in epithelial cells, which are required for cell–cell contact and cell communication, thereby establishing a coherent epithelial tissue and regulating tissue growth. The ABCP regulators are the Scribble, Par and Crumbs polarity modules [3,9]. We define these as modules rather than complexes, since although well-defined physical interactions occur between proteins of the Par and Crumbs polarity modules, it is less clear for the Scribble polarity module. The Scribble polarity module is composed of Scrib (Scribble), Dlg (discs large) and Lgl (lethal giant larvae), the Par complex is composed of Par-3, Par-6 and aPKC (atypical protein kinase C), and the Crumbs complex is composed of the transmembrane protein Crumbs, Pals and Patj (Pals1-associated tight junction protein).

In addition, to ABCP there are other forms of cell polarity. PCP (planar cell polarity) is polarity across the plane of an epithelium and refers to the ability of cells or tissues to orient in a given direction, e.g. the organization of the hair cells within the cochlea [5]. Front–rear cell polarity is important for migration, which occurs at both the level of individual cells, for example T-cell migration, and as sheets of cells, for example wound healing [4]. Finally, ACD (asymmetric cell division) refers to the ability of cells to produce two daughter cells with different cell fates and is a common process in development and in immune responses [6].

In the present chapter we focus on the Scribble polarity module. We take a historical perspective, describing the identification and biological functions of Scrib, Dlg and Lgl, as well as highlighting recent advances in our understanding of the function of the Scribble polarity module in development and cancer. We highlight the physiological function of the Scribble polarity module in different forms of cell polarity, as well as other cellular processes, including regulation of the actin cytoskeleton, cell signalling and vesicular trafficking. Furthermore, we describe how Scrib, Dlg or Lgl are altered in cancer.

The Scribble polarity module is highly conserved in evolution

Scrib, Dlg and Lgl were originally identified in the vinegar (fruit) fly *Drosophila melanogaster* by virtue of their tumorigenic mutant phenotype [10,11]. Scrib was so-called because of the disorganized epithelial phenotype observed by the mutant, Dlg was named due to the overgrowth of imaginal discs (the tissues that give rise to the *Drosophila* adult structures such as the eye and the wing) and Lgl was named because of the formation of overgrown larvae due to the inability of larval tissues to cease proliferation and differentiate. Homozygous mutants in any of the genes results in loss of ABCP and tissue overgrowth [12–15]. Since differentiation is blocked and tissue morphology is aberrant, these tumours are termed neoplastic. Indeed, genetic analysis in the *Drosophila* embryo revealed that Scrib, Dlg and Lgl function in a common pathway to regulate the establishment and maintenance of ABCP in epithelial cells [16]. Subsequently, homologues of Scrib, Dlg and Lgl have been identified in many multicellular organisms ranging from worms to man (see Table 1). There is a single mammalian homologue of Scrib (hScrib, Scrb1), four Dlgs, Dlg1 (hDlg, SAP97), Dlg2 (Chapsyn-110, PSD-93), Dlg3 (NE-Dlg, SAP102) and Dlg4 (PSD-95, SAP90), and two Lgls, Lgl1 and 2 (Hugl1 and 2) [3,9,17].

Scrib belongs to the LAP family, which describes proteins that contain either one or four PDZ [PSD (postsynaptic density)-95/Dlg/ZO (zona occludens)-1] domains and 16 LRRs (leucine-rich repeats) and function in controlling cell shape, size and subcellular protein localization [18]. Scrib contains four PDZ domains (see Figure 1), which are regions of 80–90 amino acids, found ubiquitously across the animal kingdom, and act through protein–protein interactions. LRR domains are believed to act in signalling and other LRR-domain-containing proteins, e.g. SUR-8, have been shown to interact with Ras members through their LRR domain [19]. The PDZ and LRR domains of Scrib are required for efficient activity, e.g. in correct localization and targeting to the membrane (see

Table 1. Polarity protein homologues across various species

Polarity complex	D. melanogaster (vinegar fly)	Vertebrate (other aliases)	C. elegans (worm)	D. rerio (zebrafish)
Scribble complex	Scrib	Scribble (hScrib, Scrib1, Vartul)	Let-413	Scrib (Scribble1)
	Dlg	Dlg1 (SAP97, hDlg)	Dlg-1	Dlg1 (SAP-97A)
		Dlg2 (PSD-93, Chapsyn-110)		Dlg2 (PSD-93)
		Dlg3 (SAP102, NE-Dlg)		Dlg3
		Dlg4 (PSD-95, SAP90)		Dlg4 (PSD/ SAP90)
	Lgl	Lgl1 (HUGL1, LLGL1)	Lgl (LGL-1)	Llgl1
		Lgl2 (HUGL1, LLGL2)		Llgl2 (Penner)
Par complex	Bazooka	Par3 (ASIP, PARD3)	Par-3	Pard3
	Par 6	Par6 α, β and γ (PARD6 A,B and G)	Par-6	Pard6 α, β γa and γb
	aPKC	PKCι and ζ (PKCI and 2)	PKC-3	Prkci [heart and soul (has)]
Crumbs complex	Crb	Crb1	Crb-1	Crb1
		Crb2		Crb2 α and β
		Crb3		Crb3 α and β
	Stardust	PALS1 (MPP5)	Tag-117 (C01B7.4)	Mpp5 α and β
		PALS2 (MPP6, VAM-1)		Mpp6 α and β
	Patj	PATJ (INADL)		Inadl
		MUPP1 (MPDZ)	Mpz-1 (C52A11.4)	Mpdz (Mupp1)

the section on ABCP regulation). The LRR domain is critical for function, since *Drosophila* Scrib LRR domain mutants have similar phenotypes to the complete loss of Scrib protein; however, when overexpressed, a Scrib mutant lacking the PDZ domains can function similarly to the wild-type gene *in vivo* [20].

Dlg belongs to the MAGUK (membrane-associated guanylate kinase) superfamily, which are characterized by the presence of PDZ domains, an SH3 (Src homology 3) domain and a GUK (guanylate kinase-like) domain (see Figure 1). The MAGUK family act as scaffolding proteins and are important in tethering membrane structures, adhesion and in signalling [21]. The SH3 domain is so-named due to the discovery of a homologous region in the tyrosine product of the v-Src oncogene. Although SH3 domains are not catalytic, they have been shown to couple substrates to enzymes, thereby orchestrating their enzymatic activity [22]. The GUK domains in MAGUKs are catalytically inactive due to the absence of an ATP-binding site. The MAGUK GUK domain originated

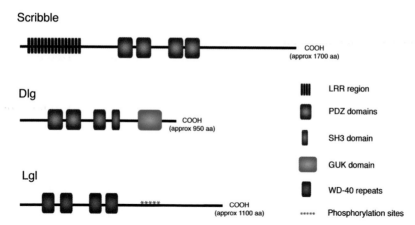

Figure 1. Schematic representation of the core members of the Scribble complex
Scribble is a LAP protein consisting of 16 LRRs and four PDZ domains. Dlg belongs to the MAGUK family and contains three PDZ domains, an SH3 domain and a GUK domain. Lgl contains several WD-40 repeats and conserved phosphorylation sites. Each of the polarity proteins are structurally highly conserved from worms through to mammals. aa, amino acids.

from a catalytically active guanylate kinase domain and gradually lost enzymatic function during evolution [23]. It is now believed that the MAGUK GUK domain functions through interactions with the SH3 domain and by interacting with proteins associated with the actin cytoskeleton and/or microtubules [24,25].

Lgl contains several WD-40 repeats (also called WD or β-transduction repeats) and conserved phosphorylation sites (see Figure 1). WD-40 repeats are structural motifs composed of approximately 40 amino acids that are named because they usually terminate in a tryptophan–aspartic acid (WD) dipeptide. WD-40 repeats function in a wide variety of processes including signal transduction, vesicle trafficking, cytoskeleton assembly and cell division [26]. The specific function of particular proteins is determined by the sequences flanking the WD-40 repeats. The WD-40 motif in Lgl has similar characteristics to those of cell-adhesion proteins [27].

Biological processes regulated by Scrib, Dlg and Lgl

Mutations in *Drosophila scrib*, *dlg* or *lgl* result in tumours in epithelial tissues, characterized by a loss in ABCP, differentiation and proliferation control, indicating that these proteins regulate tissue architecture and act as tumour suppressors [1]. Similar phenotypes are exhibited by mutation of these genes in other organisms, although the effects vary and are tissue-specific, perhaps due to redundancy with other genes.

In *Drosophila* mutants of *scrib*, *dlg* or *lgl*, apical proteins are mislocalized basolaterally and the adherens junctions do not form a tight band to form the zonula adherens, which are necessary for forming tight connections between epithelial cells and epithelial tissue architecture [15,16]. *Drosophila* Scrib, Dlg and Lgl also have roles in ACD and differentiation of the neural stem cells (neuroblasts) [6]. In addition, *Drosophila* Scrib and Lgl have been implicated in PCP [5], since they show genetic and physical interactions with core PCP regulators [28–30]. Finally, Lgl, Scrib and Dlg also have roles in cell migration of the *Drosophila* ovarian border cells; however, whereas *lgl* or *dlg* mutants increase border cell migration, *scrib* mutants inhibit it [31–33].

In the worm *Caenorhabditis elegans*, Dlg-1 or the Scrib homologue Let-413 are required for adherens junction formation [34,35]. However, in contrast with *Drosophila*, *C. elegans* Dlg-1 and Scrib appear to have distinct functions; Let-413-deficient embryos have defects in ABCP, whereas Dlg-1-deficient embryos are defective in recruitment of an adherens junction protein, AJM-1 [36,37]. The *C. elegans* Lgl homologue also has distinct functions to Dlg-1 and Let-413. Lgl functions redundantly with another cell polarity regulator, Par-2, in the maintenance of cell polarity in the early embryo [38,39].

In zebrafish, mutations in Lgl2 (Pannier) result in a failure to form hemidesmosomes (the connection between apical and basal surfaces of cells in multilayered epithelia, such as the skin) and tissue integrity of the basal epidermis [40]. By contrast, Scrib (Scribble1) has a role in PCP and cell migration [41,42].

In mammalian cells it appears that Dlg and Scrib have similar functions in cell polarity, but their requirement appears to be context-dependent. Knockdown of Dlg1 in the Caco-2 intestinal epithelial cells results in reduced accumulation of E-cadherin at the adherens junctions [43]. By contrast, Scrib knockdown does not perturb ABCP in MCF10A breast epithelial cells [44], but in SK-CO15 intestinal epithelial cells Scrib functions in the assembly of tight junctions [45]. However, Scrib has a role in directed epithelial cell migration *in vitro* and in the mouse epidermis [46]. Consistent with this, Scrib mutant mice have severe neural tube closure defects [47–49] and neural migration defects [42]. In the mouse Dlg1 also has a predominant role in epithelial migration, as evidenced by the Dlg1 mutant defects in craniofacial [50] and urogenital tract development [51]. Dlg1 is not essential for adherens junction formation, but is required for tight junction formation [52]. Lgl acts distinctly from Dlg and Scrib in mammalian cells. Lgl1-knockout mice show brain dysplasia, owing to defects in ACD and differentiation [53]. Lgl2-knockout mice exhibit branching morphogenesis defects in the placenta, which is considered to be a PCP and cell migration defect [54].

The mechanism of Scrib/Dlg/Lgl function

Regulation of cell polarity
ABCP regulation
In *Drosophila* epithelial cells, Scrib, Dlg and Lgl are localized to the cortex, basal to the adherens junction, at the septate (basolateral) junctions, and the plasma membrane localization of each protein depends on the function of the others [15]. Mammalian Scrib and Dlg are co-localized to the adherens junctions and extend basally [55,56]. In *Drosophila* the Scrib LRR region is important for

plasma membrane localization, whereas the PDZ domains of Scrib are important for recruitment to the junctional complex in epithelial cells and neuroblasts [9,20,57]. Indeed, the role of the LRR domain of Scrib in localization is evolutionarily conserved, since point mutations in the LRR domain of mouse and the worm *C. elegans* Scrib (Let-413) result in abnormal protein localization [46,58,59]. Moreover, structure–function analysis of human Scrib has revealed that both LRR and PDZ domains are required for correct localization [56,60]. PDZ domains have also been shown to be required for the correct localization of *Drosophila* Dlg [61].

Key to the regulation of ABCP is the mutual antagonism between Lgl and aPKC. The localization of Lgl is regulated by phosphorylation by aPKC (see Figure 2). Phosphorylated Lgl is unable to localize to the cortex and is inactive [9,37,62]. Mutations from serine to alanine in the aPKC phosphorylation sites of *Drosophila* or mammalian Lgl prevent it from being inactivated by aPKC phosphorylation, and the protein accumulates at the cortex [63–66] (see Figure 2a). Through binding to the Par complex, Lgl can also inhibit aPKC activity, and the defects of *Drosophila scrib*, *dlg* or *lgl* mutants can be rescued by knockdown of aPKC [67–70]. This mutual antagonism between Lgl and aPKC is evolutionarily conserved, since it is also observed in the worm, *C. elegans* [38,39], and in the frog, *Xenopus* [71]. However, in hemidesmosome formation in the zebrafish epidermis, aPKC does not seem as important as the antagonistic interaction between Lgl2 and E-cadherin [72]. The Crumbs complex also acts antagonistically to the Scrib–Dlg–Lgl complex [70,71,73]; however, the precise manner by which this regulation occurs is not known. In *Drosophila*, the Yurt–Coracle–Neurexin IV complex, and Lkb1 (liver kinase B1)-AMP-regulated protein kinase module have also been shown to regulate ABCP in some types of epithelial cells or under metabolic stress [74] (see Chapter 10); however, it is currently unknown how well conserved these modes of regulation are in other organisms.

Regulation of asymmetric cell division

In ACD of *Drosophila* neural stem cells (neuroblasts), the antagonistic relationship between Lgl and aPKC is also key (see Figure 2b). The aPKC complex is localized apically, and through the phosphorylation of Lgl, restricts Lgl from the apical cortex, thereby enabling Par (PARtitioning defective)-3 to enter the aPKC complex and promote phosphorylation of the fate-determinant Numb [63,75]. This phosphorylation of Numb is required for its asymmetric localization to the basal part of the cell during cell division and its segregation into the daughter cell (the ganglion mother cell), which is essential for differentiation. The adaptor proteins, Mira (Miranda) and Pon (partner of Numb) are required for the asymmetric localization of Numb and two other fate-determinants, Pros (Prospero) and Brat [6]. aPKC via direct phosphorylation of Mira restricts Mira to the basal cortex [76]. ACD also involves the correct orientation of the mitotic spindle in mitosis, a process co-ordinated by Insc (Inscutable), which is localized apically by binding to Par-3. Insc then recruits the NuMa [Pins (Lgn)–$G_{\alpha i}$–Mud]

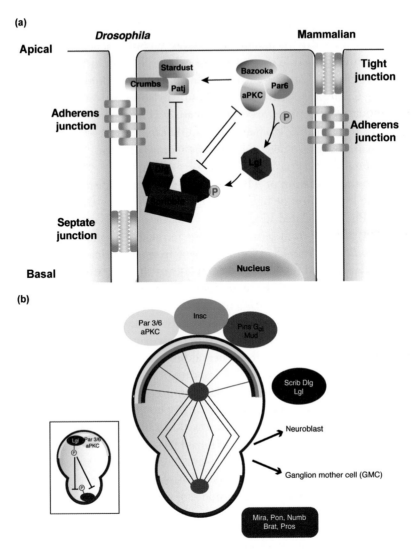

Figure 2. Models of polarity: apico–basal and asymmetric cell division
(a) Epithelial cells are polarized along their apico–basal axis through the action of three core polarity complexes. The Par complex, composed of Bazooka (Par3 in mammalian cells), Par6 and aPKC, is localized to the sub-apical domain where it promotes activity of the Crumbs complex. The Crumbs complex composed of Crumbs, Stardust (PALS1 in mammalian cells) and Patj is also localized to the apical domain. Both complexes act through mutual antagonistic interactions to maintain basolateral localization of the Scribble complex, which is composed of Scribble, Dlg and Lgl. aPKC-mediated phosphorylation of Lgl excludes it from the apical cortex and ensures that the Scribble complex remains basally located at septate junctions (equivalent to the tight junction in mammalian cells). The model illustrated here has been described in *Drosophila* and although homologues for all proteins exist in vertebrates (see Table 1), not all interactions have been formally proven in mammalian settings. (b) *Drosophila* neuroblasts are commonly used as a model for ACD. The apically located aPKC phosphorylates Lgl which in turn phosphorylates Numb. This prevents cell determinants such as Mira, Pon, Brat and Pros moving apically and ensures their segregation to the basally derived GMC (ganglion mother cell) (inset and text for further details). Insc binds to the apical Par–aPKC complex which then recruits the Pins–$G_{\alpha i}$–Mud complex. Mud binds microtubules and ensures correct spindle orientation (see text for further details).

complex, which is important for interacting with the mitotic spindle in order to correctly orientate the segregation of chromosomes during mitosis [6]. Dlg plays a different role to Lgl in ACD; it is required as a fail-safe mechanism, termed telophase rescue, to correctly align the mitotic spindle with the apical cortex via its binding to Pins [77]. Scrib shows a similar localization to Dlg in neuroblasts [78], although its precise role has not been defined. Mutations in Lgl, Dlg or Scrib show similar defects in neuroblast ACD; they exhibit defects in basal-determinant targeting, leading to symmetric divisions and an expansion of the neuroblast numbers and brain tumours [78–81]. Whether these mechanisms also occur in mammalian cells remains to be investigated; however, in the mouse skin and brain, the Pins homologue Lgn plays an important role in ACD [82,83].

Regulation of PCP
In addition to ABCP, it is becoming clear that PCP can control co-ordinated cell behaviour and is required for normal organ formation [84]. Extensive work has shown that the PCP pathway regulates the establishment of polarity within the plane of an epithelium, orthogonal to the axis of ABCP (see Figure 3a). In addition to regulating the patterning of external epidermal structures, such as wing and abdominal hair cells in *Drosophila* [85], the PCP pathway is more widely used for modifying cellular direction and movement of groups of cells, which is important for the formation of various tissues [86]. Formation of three-dimensional organs, such as the mammalian lung or kidney, requires co-ordinated behaviour across groups of cells to direct tissue morphogenesis. PCP is one such behaviour critical for organ formation, since uniform polarity across groups of cells underlies many basic cellular processes, including directional migration and orientated cell division. Disruption of PCP can lead to developmental defects, which in mammals include deafness, neural tube, heart and lung defects, and polycystic kidney disease [87,88].

The end result of the PCP pathway is polarization of the cytoskeleton, mediated by downstream effectors, which, in turn drives cellular morphogenesis and/or morphogenetic movement such as convergent extension, a process whereby cells intercalate between each other to drive tissue elongation along a particular axis. Convergent extension was originally observed in neurulation and gastrulation of the early embryo [89–91], but more recently is known to be required in various other tissues, including the mammalian cochlea [92] and kidney [93]. The downstream effector molecules of the PCP signalling pathway, including the small Rho family GTPases, RhoA, Rac1, Cdc42 (cell division cycle 42), the Rho effector ROCK (Rho-associated kinase), and the ROCK target myosin II, have all been described as PCP effectors during gastrulation of the early embryo. In addition, Rac1 mediates the polarization and morphogenesis of hair cells in the mouse inner ear, and myosin II is implicated in convergent extension of the cochlea [92].

Two parallel pathways, the 'core' PCP complex and the Fat/Dachous system can influence planar polarity. We will focus only on the 'core' PCP pathway.

(a)

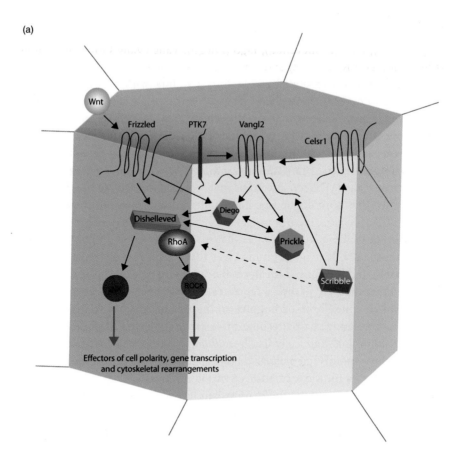

(b)

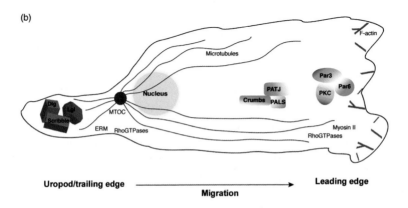

Figure 3. (Continued)

In flies, six proteins have been identified to operate within this 'core' pathway: Fz (Frizzled), Dsh (Dishevelled), Dgo (Diego), Vang (Vang Gogh, also known as Strabismus), PK (Prickle) and Fmi (Flamingo, also known as Starry-night). Complete loss of any of these proteins leads to a loss of PCP, a requirement for a protein to be considered part of the core cassette [5]. However, in vertebrates, the system is more complex due to the presence of homologues of a number of the core genes, including Frizzled, Dishevelled, Vangl and Celsr (the homologue of *Drosophila* Fmi). In addition, vertebrate genes do not always behave in the same manner as their *Drosophila* homologues. For example, overexpression of the *Drosophila* Otk (Off-track) results in defects in PCP [94], whereas loss of PTK7 (protein tyrosine kinase 7, the mammalian homologue of *Drosophila* Otk) results in identical phenotypes as core PCP mouse mutants. PTK7 has also been shown to genetically interact with core components of the PCP pathway, such as Vangl2 [95,96].

In mouse development, a clear role for Scrib has been revealed in the regulation of PCP, rather than in ABCP [47,97,98]. For example, Scrib mouse mutants exhibit classic PCP phenotypes, such as craniorachischisis, the most severe form of failed neural tube closure [47], as well as disruption to the polarity of inner ear hair cells [97]. Moreover, Vangl2, a core component of the PCP pathway, and Scrib show co-localized expression patterns and have strong genetic interactions [95,99]. In addition, Celsr1, Vangl2, Scrib and PTK7 are all required for the normal development of branched organs, including the lung [96,100]. Scrib along with Vangl2 and Celsr1 have been shown to operate via RhoA to modulate the actin–myosin cytoskeleton required for the formation and growth of new airway branches.

Figure 3. Models of polarity: planar cell polarity and migration
(a) This schematic diagram represents a simplified view of the PCP signalling pathway. The diagram shows the complex interactions between the core components of this signalling cascade. Interactions between the multiprotein complexes Celsr1–Vangl2–Prickle and Celsr1–Frizzled–Dishevelled establish planar polarity between neighbouring cells. The asymmetrical localization of these multiprotein complexes in an epithelial sheet directs cytoskeletal reorganization that allows a single hair to emerge solely from the distal edge of a cell. This same mechanism is used to direct cell movement and migration during convergent extension. During PCP signalling, Frizzled, Vangl2, Celsr1, PTK7, Prickle and Diego all signal via the cytoplasmic Dishevelled, activating downstream effector molecules, such as RhoA, ROCK and JNK (c-Jun N-terminal kinase), resulting in gene transcription, cytoskeletal remodelling and the establishment of polarity. Scribble interacts with Vangl2 and Celsr1, as well as modulating downstream effectors to regulate the establishment of PCP. (b) Cell migration requires the asymmetric localization of polarity molecules to opposite sides of the cell. Using T-cell migration as an example, this schematic diagram depicts how the Par complex is located to the front of the migrating cell and the Scribble complex towards the uropod at the rear of the cell. The precise location of the Crumbs complex is still to be determined, but current research suggests that it sits between the Par and Scribble complexes. The microtubule-organizing centre (MTOC) is required for the contractile motions that drive T-cell migration. Rho GTPases play key roles in uropod formation, through interactions with ERM (erzin/radixin/moesin) and by mediating the actomyosin cytoskeleton at the leading edge.

While the majority of studies indicate the Scribble polarity module to have a role in ABCP in *Drosophila* and PCP in mammalian systems, more recently a role for Scrib in establishing PCP in *Drosophila* [28], and in ABCP in mammary and prostate epithelial cells [101,102] has been determined. Moreover, studies in zebrafish, revealed that Scrib is required for convergent extension of mesenchymal cells [41], which lack ABCP, suggesting additional functions for Scrib in PCP patterning. Indeed, *Drosophila* studies show that PCP and ABCP pathways are closely linked at the molecular level [28,103]. Furthermore, the PCP protein Dsh binds to Lgl and regulates its localization in *Drosophila* epithelium and frog (*Xenopus*) tissues [30]. Thus it is likely that many epithelial tissues require both ABCP and planar polarization for optimal organization and function, and the Scribble polarity module may be the link between these two polarity pathways.

Regulation of directed cell migration

Another role that has been attributed to the Scribble polarity module and components of the PCP pathway is the regulation of directed migration of cells and vertebrate wound healing. PCP signalling results in the reorganization and polarization of the actin cytoskeleton and subcellular organelles at the leading edge of tissues, such as that which occurs when the skin is wounded, so that keratinocytes (skin epithelial cells) can undergo co-ordinated cell movement from the wound edge to close the gap [104]. Scrib has been shown to be essential for proper epithelial cell movements in response to extracellular directional migration cues during wound healing [46]. Scrib co-localizes with Rac and Cdc42 at the leading edge of migrating cells and is required for the recruitment of these GTPases to this site. Furthermore, this function of Scrib in regulating cell migration is conserved between different epithelial cell types and species, as mutational disruption of Scrib function in the mouse results in defective wound healing of the epidermis *in vivo* [46]. A more recent study confirmed the role of Scrib in effective wound healing in the mouse and implicated both Celsr1 and the vertebrate PCP component PTK7 in this process [95,104]. Dlg1 is also required for epithelial cell migration during mouse embryogenesis, with loss-of-function mutants resulting in craniofacial defects [50], and epithelial duct formation and morphogenesis defects in urogenital development [51].

Scrib can also control the migration of non-epithelial cell types, such as zebrafish motor neurons, mouse astrocytes and T-lymphocytes, by regulating front–rear polarity [41,105,106]. Here we will focus on T-lymphocytes. T-cell shape is determined by the selective polarized recruitment of molecules to different regions of the cell and is crucial for T-cell function, from migration to cell killing. Scrib and other polarity proteins (Lgl, Par3 and Crumbs) are expressed in T-cells and are thought to be critical for their function (see Figure 3b). As with other migrating cells [4,107], the opposing action of the Scribble polarity module with the Par and Crumbs complexes is also thought to be important for T-cell front–rear polarity and migration. Indeed, knockdown of Scrib in murine

T-lymphocytes results in a profound defect in cell polarity and loss of directed cell migration [105]. Whether Dlg or Lgl also function in this manner in T-cells is more difficult to discern due to the presence of multiple family members (see Table 1).

In summary, the Scribble polarity module plays a central role in different forms of cell polarity, ABCP, ACD, PCP and front–rear, in different cell types. An important theme to emerge from these studies is that Scrib, Dlg and Lgl often have distinct roles, and therefore cannot always be considered as working in a common pathway. Key questions still remaining are what are the precise mechanisms by which Scrib, Dlg and Lgl function to control these different types of polarity and how do other cellular processes that are regulated by these proteins [such as actin remodelling, cell signalling and vesicular trafficking (see below)] connect to cell polarity regulation?

Regulation of the actin cytoskeleton by Scrib, Dlg and Lgl

The regulation of cell polarity involves remodelling of the actin cytoskeleton; however, at present only sketchy details have been revealed on the molecular mechanism by which Scrib, Dlg or Lgl mediate this regulation. As described above, there are links via PCP proteins to the Rho-GTPase family of actin regulators, and in cell migration Scrib has been connected to Rac-GTPase regulation, via binding to and controlling its regulators, β-Pix and Git1 [108,109]. Recently another actin regulator connecting Scrib and Dlg to the actin cytoskeleton has emerged, Gukh. Gukh (NHS) is an evolutionarily conserved protein identified as tethering Dlg and Scrib together in *Drosophila* neuromuscular junctions [110,111]. NHS is mutated in the human developmental disorder Nance–Horan Syndrome, and is involved in remodelling the actin cytoskeleton and cell morphology in mammalian cells [112]. This role of NHS is likely to be important in linking Scrib to the regulation of PCP and cell migration [42].

Lgl appears to regulate the actin cytoskeleton differently. Lgl binds to and negatively regulates the non-muscle myosin protein, myosin II, a regulator of F-actin (filamentous actin) function in cell morphology regulation, in *Drosophila* and human cells [113–115]. Recently evidence has emerged that, in *Drosophila*, this regulation may play an important role in PCP [29], although the role of this interaction in *Drosophila* ABCP or ACD is unclear [29,76]. However, in *C. elegans*, Lgl-1 negatively regulates the accumulation of myosin II (NMY-2) on the posterior cortex of the early embryo in the establishment of ABCP [39]. In this system, the myosin II-mediated contraction of cortical F-actin, asymmetrically distributes PAR-3, PAR-6 and aPKC (PKC-3) to the anterior. Thus, in the worm embryo, Lgl seems to play an important role in ABCP through its regulation of myosin II as well as aPKC.

Regulation of signalling pathways by Scrib, Dlg and Lgl

The Scribble polarity module has been linked to the regulation of many signalling pathways that play critical roles in cell growth, proliferation and survival [1].

Here we highlight important new insights that have emerged for Scrib, Dlg and Lgl in regulating signalling pathways involved in tissue growth control.

In *Drosophila*, a role for Lgl in cell proliferation and survival has been uncovered, which is separable from its role in ABCP [116]. By making mutant patches of tissue in the developing *Drosophila* eye, the G_1–S-phase cell-cycle regulator cyclin E and the cell-cycle transcription factor E2F1 were shown to be ectopically expressed, in a region of the developing eye where cells have normally exited from the cell cycle. Moreover, the cell death inhibitor Diap1 (*Drosophila* inhibitor of apoptosis) is up-regulated and developmental cell death blocked [68,116]. This up-regulation of cyclin E, E2F1 and Diap1 is due to the inhibition of the Hippo negative tissue growth control pathway. The evolutionarily conserved Hippo signalling pathway consists of a kinase cascade involving the Hippo and Warts protein kinases that phosphorylate and inactivate the Yorkie [YAP (Yes-associated protein)/TAZ (transcriptional coactivator with PDZ-binding motif) in mammalian cells] transcriptional co-activator [117] (see Chapter 9). This finding that loss-of-function of Lgl (and up-regulation of aPKC) inactivates Hippo pathway signalling [thereby leading to increased expression of Yorkie targets, including tissue growth genes such as *CCNE1* (*cyclin E*), *E2F1* and *Diap1*], has provided a link between Lgl/aPKC balance and regulation of tissue growth via Hippo pathway regulation in *Drosophila* [68,118,119]. The mechanism by which Lgl/aPKC regulates the Hippo pathway is currently unclear; however, deregulation of Hippo signalling correlates with delocalization of the Hippo protein kinase from the apical membrane, where it normally functions [120,121]. Interestingly, depleting Scrib or Dlg does not lead to deregulation of Hippo pathway signalling unless ABCP is lost [68,122]. A possible mechanism by which Scrib may control the Hippo pathway has been revealed by a recent study showing that mammalian Scrib can bind to TAZ (the positive transcriptional co-activator that is negatively regulated by Hippo pathway signalling) and sequester it to the cell cortex in breast cancer stem cells [123]. Therefore, when Scrib or ABCP is lost, TAZ would be expected to be released from the cortex and function as a transcriptional co-activator. Whether this control extends to other cell types or other organisms remains to be determined. Another mechanism by which Scrib deregulation could result in Hippo pathway deregulation is via its effect on E-cadherin; in MDCK kidney epithelial cells, loss of Scribble destabilizes the coupling between E-cadherin and α-catenin and results in decreased adhesion [4]. Since α-catenin restricts Hippo pathway signalling by tethering YAP to the cortex [124,125], then knock down of Scrib would be expected to release YAP from the cell cortex enabling it to enter the nucleus to activate transcription of tissue growth genes. Furthermore, depletion of Scrib in *Drosophila* results in increased F-actin accumulation, which has been shown to reduce Hippo pathway signalling and increase tissue growth [126,127]. Loss of polarity induced by Scrib or Dlg depletion would also lead to expansion of the apical domain and higher levels of aPKC and Crumbs that could also contribute to Hippo pathway inactivation [68,118]. In development and tissue homoeostasis, Lgl/aPKC balance, and perhaps also Scrib and Dlg, may relay cues from the surrounding cells and the microenvironment to regulate the Hippo tissue growth control pathway, thereby modulating cell proliferation, survival and differentiation. Indeed, in zebrafish, Scrib has been linked to Hippo pathway regulation in pronephros development [128].

Scrib has also been implicated in the EGFR (epidermal growth factor receptor)-Ras GTPase signalling pathway to control cell proliferation and survival in both mammalian cells and *Drosophila* [44,129]. The EGFR-Ras signalling pathway signals through a kinase cascade involving Raf, MEK [MAPK (mitogen-activated protein kinase)/ERK (extracellular-signal-regulated kinase) kinase] and MAPK (ERK), to promote proliferation and survival, and is one of the major pathways deregulated in human cancers [130]. In mammalian cells, Scrib functions as a scaffolding protein for Ras signalling; it binds to MAPK (ERK) through a conserved domain, KIM (kinase-interaction motif) [129]. However, it is likely that there are additional tiers of regulation of Ras-MAPK signalling by Scrib, for example Scrib can also interact with RSK2 (ribosomal S6 kinase 2), a negative regulator of the pathway [131], and GIT1 [G-protein-coupled receptor kinase-interacting Arf (ADP-ribosylation factor)-GAP (GTPase-activating protein) 1], an Arf-GAP that can act as a MEK-ERK scaffold [132,133]. Interestingly, in zebrafish, Lgl2 has also been linked to regulation of the Ras signalling pathway [134]; however, how direct this is and whether this regulation also occurs in other organisms remains to be determined.

The Scribble polarity module can also have an impact on the regulation of the PI3K (phosphoinositide 3-kinase) pathway. The PI3K pathway is regulated at adherens junctions and acts via the protein kinases, Akt and TOR (target of rapamycin), leading to up-regulation of translation and thereby cell growth and proliferation, as well as promoting cell survival [135,136]. In mammalian cells, Dlg1 has been shown to bind to PTEN (phosphatase and tensin homologue deleted on chromosome 10), a negative regulator of the PI3K pathway [137], and Dlg1 is required for the Adenovirus 9 E4-ORF1 (*E4* region-encoded open reading frame 1) oncoprotein to promote the constitutive activation of PI3K [138]. Consistent with a role for Dlg in promoting PI3K signalling, a recent study in *Drosophila* showed that PI3K signalling is down-regulated in Dlg-depleted epithelial cells, and further knockdown of PI3K components resulted in synthetic lethality of Dlg-depleted tissue, even in the presence of oncogenic Ras [139]. Conversely, in mammalian cells, Scrib negatively regulates Akt activity via binding to Phlpp [PH (pleckstrin homology) domain and LRR protein phosphatase], a protein phosphatase that negatively regulates Akt, and localizes it to the plasma membrane [140]. Scrib forms a tripartite complex with Phlpp and Akt, thereby inhibiting Akt activity, but when Scrib is down-regulated, Phlpp is released, Akt activity is increased and cell growth, proliferation and survival is enhanced.

In summary, the common theme emerging from these studies is that the Scribble polarity module proteins may serve as signalling scaffolds controlling many signalling pathways, but which signalling pathways are regulated in specific cells or organisms may be context-dependent.

Regulation of vesicular trafficking by Scrib, Dlg and Lgl

In *Drosophila*, neoplastic tumour phenotypes are also observed in mutants affecting endocytosis, the process by which external and membrane-bound proteins are trafficked into a cell [141]. There is accumulating evidence for the role of vesicular trafficking in the localization of cell polarity proteins; however, the ABCP machinery can also control vesicular trafficking [142]. The Par complex has been implicated in endocytosis regulation from a genetic screen in *C. elegans* [143]. Furthermore, in *Drosophila* epithelial tissues, mutants in Par complex proteins exhibit defects in E-cadherin trafficking [144,145], and in endocytosis of apical proteins [146]. In mammalian cells, Scrib inhibits basal receptor endocytosis and promotes recycling of the TSHR (thyroid-stimulating hormone receptor) in PC12 cells [108].

Exocytosis, the trafficking of proteins after protein synthesis in the endoplasmic reticulum to the plasma membrane [147], has also been linked to the Scribble polarity module. In *Drosophila*, *scrib*, *dlg* and *lgl* genetically interact with mutants in a core component of the exocytic machinery, *exo84*, which is required for the apical delivery of proteins [148]. In MDCK (Madin–Darby canine kidney) mammalian epithelial cells, Lgl2 forms a complex with the t-SNARE [target SNARE (soluble *N*-ethylmaleimide-sensitive fusion protein-attachment protein receptor)] syntaxin 4, a component of the basolateral exocyst machinery [149], which parallels studies in yeast where the Lgl homologues Sro7 and Sro77 interact with the exocytic machinery [150,151]. Furthermore, in response to osmotic stress, syntaxin 4 forms a complex with Scrib, Dlg and Lgl and is required for their membrane localization [152]. Lgl1 has also been shown to interact with and regulate the small GTPase Rab10 in directional membrane insertion during mammalian axonal development [153]. Furthermore, in mammalian cells, Scrib, through its association with β-Pix and GIT1 (Rac GTPase regulators), has an important role in regulating exocytosis in neuroendocrine cells [133].

Collectively, these data suggest that members of the Scribble polarity module may be playing key roles in vesicle trafficking. Since many signalling pathways involve vesicle trafficking to promote signalling, or to down-regulate receptors and dampen signalling [154], this connection of Scrib–Dlg–Lgl to vesicle trafficking may be fundamental to their regulation of signalling pathways. Although this field is still in its infancy, distinct roles for Scrib, Dlg and Lgl in specific aspects of vesicular trafficking are being revealed. Future research will need to focus on discerning the universality of each of these mechanisms and how they relate to effects of Scrib, Dlg or Lgl on cell polarity, signalling pathways or actin cytoskeletal regulation.

Role of Scrib/Dlg/Lgl in cancer progression and metastasis

Since the original identification of Scrib, Dlg and Lgl as neoplastic tumour suppressors in *Drosophila*, much effort has focused on understanding their involvement in mammalian cancer progression and metastasis. We describe below evidence revealing an important role for the Scribble polarity module in mammalian cancer.

Scrib and Dlg are targets of viral oncoproteins

Over 80% of cervical cancers are caused by the high-risk human papilloma viruses HPV16 and HPV18, which target PDZ-domain-containing proteins for degradation via the E6 oncoprotein [155]. Several polarity proteins contain PDZ domains, including Scrib, Dlg1, MAGI-1 (membrane-associated guanylate kinase, WW and PDZ domain-containing protein 1) and MUPP1 (multi-PDZ-domain protein 1), and have been identified as targets of the E6 oncoprotein [155–159]. Importantly, the transforming capacity of the E6 oncoprotein is dependent on direct interaction with PDZ proteins, as mutants that lack the PDZ-binding motif no longer transform cells [160].

In addition to HPV16 and HPV18, several other human tumour viruses have been identified in which their oncogenic potential depends, in part, on their ability to inactivate polarity proteins. Adenovirus type 9 promotes transformation through E4-ORF1 via interactions with the polarity proteins Dlg1, MUPP1, PATJ and ZO (zona occludens)-2 [157,158,161,162]. HTLV-1 (human T-cell leukaemia virus type 1) Tax oncoproteins are causative agents for adult T-cell leukaemia and have been shown to target the polarity proteins Dlg and Scrib [162,163]. The role of polarity deregulation in tumorigenesis has primarily focused on epithelial tumours, however, the ability of Adenovirus 9 and HTLV-1 to promote sarcomas and leukaemias respectively, supports a wider role for polarity deregulation in the development of many cancer types [164].

Aberrant expression of Scrib, Dlg and Lgl in human cancer

Consolidated analysis from both primary tissue samples and cell lines suggests that altered expression of polarity proteins play a causal role in tumorigenesis [165]. All three members of the Scribble polarity module are mislocalized in various human cancers. A recent study found Scrib mislocalized in 50% of analysed DCIS (ductal carcinoma *in situ*) breast cancer lesions, and Scrib and Dlg has been shown to be mislocalized in colon and cervical cancer, whereas Lgl2 is mislocalized in gastric adenocarcinomas [101,166–168]. Members of the Scribble polarity module frequently show aberrant expression across a variety of tumour types, including breast, endometrial, cervical, colon, prostate and lung [101,102,166–172]. Altered expression patterns of other polarity complexes, for example the Par complex, are also seen in several tumour types, including breast, oesophaegeal and ovarian carcinomas [173–176]. Furthermore, enforced expression in transformed cell lines of polarity proteins, including

Scrib, Lgl and Crumbs3, results in an increase in cell adhesion and reversion to a less malignant phenotype, suggestive of a direct role for polarity regulators in tumour progression [44,177–179]. Taken together, these studies support the idea that aberrant expression of polarity proteins correlates with malignancy and invasion, although direct links to clinical outcome remain to be established. To bridge this gap, researchers are developing *in vivo* mouse models to investigate the consequences of polarity deregulation in tumorigenesis.

In vivo models of Scrib, Dlg and Lgl knockdown in tumorigenesis

Scrib, unlike other members of the complex, has a single homologue (see Table 1), enabling it to be studied without the complicating factors of redundancy. Mice that have lost both copies of Scrib die perinatally, however, analysis of heterozygous mice enables the study of the effects of reduced Scrib expression. Aged Scrib$^{+/-}$ mice show prostate hyperplasia and have a high incidence of lung adenomas [102]. The effect of Scrib depletion has also been analysed by transplantation of epithelial cells in which Scrib was knocked down [using RNAi (RNA interference)] into the mouse mammary fat pad; Scrib-depleted tissues exhibit multilayering and eventually a small percentage develop tumours [101]. Similar to studies in *Drosophila,* where mutants in *scrib*, *dlg* and *lgl* co-operate in tumorigenesis with various oncogenes, such as Myc and Ras [180,181], the Myc oncogene also co-operates with Scrib depletion to promote tumorigenesis in mouse xenograft models [101]. Co-operation between Scrib and the Ras oncogene also occurs in other settings, such as the prostate [102], suggesting that such co-operation may be a conserved phenomenon.

Conclusions and future perspectives

As outlined in the present chapter, the Scribble polarity module has roles in a plethora of biological processes. In the years since the initial discovery of Scrib, Dlg and Lgl [12,14,15], we have learnt that their functions are far more extensive than the roles in ABCP, junctional integrity and cell proliferation for which they were originally identified. It is now clear that they play roles in the regulation of other types of polarity, the actin cytoskeleton, cell signalling and vesicle trafficking. The context-dependent roles that Scrib, Dlg and Lgl often exhibit have complicated studies investigating their physiological functions. For the most part, the structure and function of members of the Scribble polarity module are evolutionarily well conserved, which has enabled researchers to study the proteins in simpler organisms, such as the vinegar fly *Drosophila melanogaster,* the worm *C. elegans* and the zebrafish *Danio rerio,* before translating the findings into the more complex mammalian systems. The emergence of a crucial role for Scribble polarity module proteins in cancer progression and metastasis has spurred the development of many *in vivo* models to aid in the understanding of how their deregulation contributes to tumorigenesis. Although, much progress has been made in this fascinating and ever-growing field, we still have a long way to go before fully understanding how Scrib, Dlg and Lgl function, and how they interact both among themselves and with other proteins physiologically and in tumorigenesis.

Summary

- *The Scribble polarity module comprises three evolutionarily conserved proteins, Scrib, Dlg and Lgl.*
- *Scrib, Dlg and Lgl function in the same genetic pathway in ABCP regulation.*
- *Scrib, Dlg and Lgl also have specific roles in other forms of polarity: ACD, PCP and front–rear polarity in cell migration.*
- *The Scribble polarity module regulates the actin cytoskeleton via different mechanisms.*
- *Scrib, Dlg and Lgl have distinct regulatory effects on signalling pathways that control cell growth, proliferation and survival.*
- *The regulation of vesicular trafficking via the Scribble polarity module may be key to its function in regulating signalling pathways.*
- *Deregulation of the Scribble polarity module is commonly observed in human cancer and correlates with tumour progression.*

We thank the National Heath and Medical Research Council (NHMRC) of Australia for grant support. H.E.R. is supported by an NHMRC Senior Research Fellowship and P.O.H. by an NHMRC Biomedical Career Development Award Fellowship.

References

1.   Humbert, P.O., Grzeschik, N.A., Brumby, A.M., Galea, R., Elsum, I. and Richardson, H.E. (2008) Control of tumourigenesis by the Scribble/Dlg/Lgl polarity module. Oncogene **27**, 6888–6907
2.   Bulgakova, N.A. and Knust, E. (2009) The Crumbs complex: from epithelial-cell polarity to retinal degeneration. J. Cell Sci. **122**, 2587–2596
3.   Assemat, E., Bazellieres, E., Pallesi-Pocachard, E., Le Bivic, A. and Massey-Harroche, D. (2008) Polarity complex proteins. Biochim. Biophys. Acta **1778**, 614–630
4.   Dow, L.E. and Humbert, P.O. (2007) Polarity regulators and the control of epithelial architecture, cell migration, and tumorigenesis. Int. Rev. Cytol. **262**, 253–302
5.   Goodrich, L.V. and Strutt, D. (2011) Principles of planar polarity in animal development. Development **138**, 1877–1892
6.   Knoblich, J.A. (2008) Mechanisms of asymmetric stem cell division. Cell **132**, 583–597
7.   St Johnston, D. and Sanson, B. (2011) Epithelial polarity and morphogenesis. Curr. Opin. Cell Biol. **23**, 540–546
8.   St Johnston, D. and Ahringer, J. (2010) Cell polarity in eggs and epithelia: parallels and diversity. Cell **141**, 757–774
9.   Yamanaka, T. and Ohno, S. (2008) Role of Lgl/Dlg/Scribble in the regulation of epithelial junction, polarity and growth. Front Biosci. **13**, 6693–6707
10. Gateff, E. (1994) Tumor suppressor and overgrowth suppressor genes of *Drosophila melanogaster*: developmental aspects. Int. J. Dev. Biol. **38**, 565–590

11. Hariharan, I.K. and Bilder, D. (2006) Regulation of imaginal disc growth by tumor-suppressor genes in Drosophila. Annu. Rev. Genet. **40**, 335–361

12. Woods, D.F. and Bryant, P.J. (1989) Molecular cloning of the lethal(1)discs large-1 oncogene of Drosophila. Dev. Biol. **134**, 222–235

13. Gateff, E. and Schneiderman, H.A. (1974) Developmental capacities of benign and malignant neoplasms of Drosophila. Roux's Arch. Dev. Biol. **176**, 23–65

14. Mechler, B.M., McGinnis, W. and Gehring, W.J. (1985) Molecular cloning of lethal(2)giant larvae, a recessive oncogene of Drosophila melanogaster. EMBO J. **4**, 1551–1557

15. Bilder, D. and Perrimon, N. (2000) Localization of apical epithelial determinants by the basolateral PDZ protein Scribble. Nature **403**, 676–680

16. Bilder, D., Li, M. and Perrimon, N. (2000) Cooperative regulation of cell polarity and growth by Drosophila tumor suppressors. Science **289**, 113–116

17. Humbert, P.O., Dow, L.E. and Russell, S.M. (2006) The Scribble and Par complexes in polarity and migration: friends or foes? Trends Cell Biol. **16**, 622–630

18. Bryant, P.J. and Huwe, A. (2000) LAP proteins: what's up with epithelia? Nat. Cell Biol. **2**, E141–E143

19. Sieburth, D.S., Sun, Q. and Han, M. (1998) SUR-8, a conserved Ras-binding protein with leucine-rich repeats, positively regulates Ras-mediated signaling in C. elegans. Cell **94**, 119–130

20. Zeitler, J., Hsu, C.P., Dionne, H. and Bilder, D. (2004) Domains controlling cell polarity and proliferation in the Drosophila tumor suppressor Scribble. J. Cell Biol. **167**, 1137–1146

21. Pan, L., Chen, J., Yu, J., Yu, H. and Zhang, M. (2011) The structure of the PDZ3-SH3-GuK tandem of ZO-1 protein suggests a supramodular organization of the membrane-associated guanylate kinase (MAGUK) family scaffold protein core. J. Biol. Chem. **286**, 40069–40074

22. Gonzalez-Mariscal, L., Betanzos, A. and Avila-Flores, A. (2000) MAGUK proteins: structure and role in the tight junction. Semin. Cell Dev. Biol. **11**, 315–324

23. te Velthuis, A.J., Admiraal, J.F. and Bagowski, C.P. (2007) Molecular evolution of the MAGUK family in metazoan genomes. BMC Evol. Biol. **7**, 129

24. Hanada, T., Lin, L., Tibaldi, E.V., Reinherz, E.L. and Chishti, A.H. (2000) GAKIN, a novel kinesin-like protein associates with the human homologue of the Drosophila discs large tumor suppressor in T lymphocytes. J. Biol. Chem. **275**, 28774–28784

25. Bauer, H., Zweimueller-Mayer, J., Steinbacher, P., Lametschwandtner, A. and Bauer, H.C. (2010) The dual role of zonula occludens (ZO) proteins. J. Biomed. Biotechnol. **2010**, 402593

26. Smith, T.F., Gaitatzes, C., Saxena, K. and Neer, E.J. (1999) The WD repeat: a common architecture for diverse functions. Trends Biochem. Sci. **24**, 181–185

27. Lutzelschwab, R., Klambt, C., Rossa, R. and Schmidt, O. (1987) A protein product of the Drosophila recessive tumor gene, l (2) giant gl, potentially has cell adhesion properties. EMBO J. **6**, 1791–1797

28. Courbard, J.R., Djiane, A., Wu, J. and Mlodzik, M. (2009) The apical/basal-polarity determinant Scribble cooperates with the PCP core factor Stbm/Vang and functions as one of its effectors. Dev. Biol. **333**, 67–77

29. Kaplan, N.A. and Tolwinski, N.S. (2010) Spatially defined Dsh-Lgl interaction contributes to directional tissue morphogenesis. J. Cell Sci. **123**, 3157–3165

30. Dollar, G.L., Weber, U., Mlodzik, M. and Sokol, S.Y. (2005) Regulation of Lethal giant larvae by Dishevelled. Nature **437**, 1376–1380

31. Zhao, M., Szafranski, P., Hall, C.A. and Goode, S. (2008) Basolateral junctions utilize warts signaling to control epithelial-mesenchymal transition and proliferation crucial for migration and invasion of Drosophila ovarian epithelial cells. Genetics **178**, 1947–1971

32. Szafranski, P. and Goode, S. (2007) Basolateral junctions are sufficient to suppress epithelial invasion during Drosophila oogenesis. Dev. Dyn. **236**, 364–373

33. Szafranski, P. and Goode, S. (2004) A Fasciclin 2 morphogenetic switch organizes epithelial cell cluster polarity and motility. Development **131**, 2023–2036

34. Bossinger, O., Klebes, A., Segbert, C., Theres, C. and Knust, E. (2001) Zonula adherens formation in *Caenorhabditis elegans* requires dlg-1, the homologue of the *Drosophila* gene discs large. Dev. Biol. **230**, 29–42

35. Legouis, R., Gansmuller, A., Sookhareea, S., Bosher, J.M., Baillie, D.L. and Labouesse, M. (2000) LET-413 is a basolateral protein required for the assembly of adherens junctions in *Caenorhabditis elegans*. Nat. Cell Biol. **2**, 415–422

36. McMahon, L., Legouis, R., Vonesch, J.L. and Labouesse, M. (2001) Assembly of *C. elegans* apical junctions involves positioning and compaction by LET-413 and protein aggregation by the MAGUK protein DLG-1. J. Cell Sci. **114**, 2265–2277

37. Koppen, M., Simske, J.S., Sims, P.A., Firestein, B.L., Hall, D.H., Radice, A.D., Rongo, C. and Hardin, J.D. (2001) Cooperative regulation of AJM-1 controls junctional integrity in *Caenorhabditis elegans* epithelia. Nat. Cell Biol. **3**, 983–991

38. Hoege, C., Constantinescu, A.T., Schwager, A., Goehring, N.W., Kumar, P. and Hyman, A.A. (2010) LGL can partition the cortex of one-cell *Caenorhabditis elegans* embryos into two domains. Curr. Biol. **20**, 1296–1303

39. Beatty, A., Morton, D. and Kemphues, K. (2010) The *C. elegans* homolog of *Drosophila* Lethal giant larvae functions redundantly with PAR-2 to maintain polarity in the early embryo. Development **137**, 3995–4004

40. Sonawane, M., Carpio, Y., Geisler, R., Schwarz, H., Maischein, H.M. and Nuesslein-Volhard, C. (2005) Zebrafish penner/lethal giant larvae 2 functions in hemidesmosome formation, maintenance of cellular morphology and growth regulation in the developing basal epidermis. Development **132**, 3255–3265

41. Wada, H., Iwasaki, M., Sato, T., Masai, I., Nishiwaki, Y., Tanaka, H., Sato, A., Nojima, Y. and Okamoto, H. (2005) Dual roles of zygotic and maternal Scribble1 in neural migration and convergent extension movements in zebrafish embryos. Development **132**, 2273–2285

42. Walsh, G.S., Grant, P.K., Morgan, J.A. and Moens, C.B. (2011) Planar polarity pathway and Nance-Horan syndrome-like 1b have essential cell-autonomous functions in neuronal migration. Development **138**, 3033–3042

43. Laprise, P., Viel, A. and Rivard, N. (2004) Human homolog of disc-large is required for adherens junction assembly and differentiation of human intestinal epithelial cells. J. Biol. Chem. **279**, 10157–10166

44. Dow, L.E., Elsum, I.A., King, C.L., Kinross, K.M., Richardson, H.E. and Humbert, P.O. (2008) Loss of human Scribble cooperates with H-Ras to promote cell invasion through deregulation of MAPK signalling. Oncogene **27**, 5988–6001

45. Ivanov, A.I., Young, C., Den Beste, K., Capaldo, C.T., Humbert, P.O., Brennwald, P., Parkos, C.A. and Nusrat, A. (2010) Tumor suppressor scribble regulates assembly of tight junctions in the intestinal epithelium. Am. J. Pathol. **176**, 134–145

46. Dow, L.E., Kauffman, J.S., Caddy, J., Zarbalis, K., Peterson, A.S., Jane, S.M., Russell, S.M. and Humbert, P.O. (2007) The tumour-suppressor Scribble dictates cell polarity during directed epithelial migration: regulation of Rho GTPase recruitment to the leading edge. Oncogene **26**, 2272–2282

47. Murdoch, J.N., Henderson, D.J., Doudney, K., Gaston-Massuet, C., Phillips, H.M., Paternotte, C., Arkell, R., Stanier, P. and Copp, A.J. (2003) Disruption of scribble (Scrb1) causes severe neural tube defects in the circletail mouse. Hum. Mol. Genet. **12**, 87–98

48. Wansleeben, C., van Gurp, L., Feitsma, H., Kroon, C., Rieter, E., Verberne, M., Guryev, V., Cuppen, E. and Meijlink, F. (2011) An ENU-mutagenesis screen in the mouse: identification of novel developmental gene functions. PLoS ONE **6**, e19357

49. Robinson, A., Escuin, S., Doudney, K., Vekemans, M., Stevenson, R.E., Greene, N.D., Copp, A.J. and Stanier, P. (2012) Mutations in the planar cell polarity genes CELSR1 and SCRIB are associated with the severe neural tube defect craniorachischisis. Hum. Mutat. **33**, 440–447

50. Caruana, G. and Bernstein, A. (2001) Craniofacial dysmorphogenesis including cleft palate in mice with an insertional mutation in the discs large gene. Mol. Cell. Biol. **21**, 1475–1483

51. Iizuka-Kogo, A., Ishidao, T., Akiyama, T. and Senda, T. (2007) Abnormal development of urogenital organs in Dlgl-deficient mice. Development **134**, 1799–1807

52. Stucke, V.M., Timmerman, E., Vandekerckhove, J., Gevaert, K. and Hall, A. (2007) The MAGUK protein MPP7 binds to the polarity protein hDlgl and facilitates epithelial tight junction formation. Mol. Biol. Cell **18**, 1744–1755

53. Klezovitch, O., Fernandez, T.E., Tapscott, S.J. and Vasioukhin, V. (2004) Loss of cell polarity causes severe brain dysplasia in Lgl1 knockout mice. Genes Dev. **18**, 559–571

54. Sripathy, S., Lee, M. and Vasioukhin, V. (2011) Mammalian Llgl2 is necessary for proper branching morphogenesis during placental development. Mol. Cell. Biol. **31**, 2920–2933

55. Dow, L.E., Brumby, A.M., Muratore, R., Coombe, M.L., Sedelies, K.A., Trapani, J.A., Russell, S.M., Richardson, H.E. and Humbert, P.O. (2003) hScrib is a functional homologue of the *Drosophila* tumour suppressor Scribble. Oncogene **22**, 9225–9230

56. Navarro, C., Nola, S., Audebert, S., Santoni, M.J., Arsanto, J.P., Ginestier, C., Marchetto, S., Jacquemier, J., Isnardon, D., Le Bivic, A. et al. (2005) Junctional recruitment of mammalian Scribble relies on E-cadherin engagement. Oncogene **24**, 4330–4339

57. Albertson, R., Chabu, C., Sheehan, A. and Doe, C.Q. (2004) Scribble protein domain mapping reveals a multistep localization mechanism and domains necessary for establishing cortical polarity. J. Cell Sci. **117**, 6061–6070

58. Legouis, R., Jaulin-Bastard, F., Schott, S., Navarro, C., Borg, J.P. and Labouesse, M. (2003) Basolateral targeting by leucine-rich repeat domains in epithelial cells. EMBO Rep. **4**, 1096–1102

59. Zarbalis, K., May, S.R., Shen, Y., Ekker, M., Rubenstein, J.L. and Peterson, A.S. (2004) A focused and efficient genetic screening strategy in the mouse: identification of mutations that disrupt cortical development. PLoS Biol. **2**, E219

60. Nagasaka, K., Nakagawa, S., Yano, T., Takizawa, S., Matsumoto, Y., Tsuruga, T., Nakagawa, K., Minaguchi, T., Oda, K., Hiraike-Wada, O. et al. (2006) Human homolog of *Drosophila* tumor suppressor Scribble negatively regulates cell-cycle progression from G1 to S phase by localizing at the basolateral membrane in epithelial cells. Cancer Sci. **97**, 1217–1225

61. Hough, C.D., Woods, D.F., Park, S. and Bryant, P.J. (1997) Organizing a functional junctional complex requires specific domains of the *Drosophila* MAGUK Discs large. Genes Dev. **11**, 3242–3253

62. Wirtz-Peitz, F. and Knoblich, J.A. (2006) Lethal giant larvae take on a life of their own. Trends Cell Biol. **16**, 234–241

63. Betschinger, J., Mechtler, K. and Knoblich, J.A. (2003) The Par complex directs asymmetric cell division by phosphorylating the cytoskeletal protein Lgl. Nature **422**, 326–330

64. Plant, P.J., Fawcett, J.P., Lin, D.C., Holdorf, A.D., Binns, K., Kulkarni, S. and Pawson, T. (2003) A polarity complex of mPar-6 and atypical PKC binds, phosphorylates and regulates mammalian Lgl. Nat. Cell Biol. **5**, 301–308

65. Yamanaka, T., Horikoshi, Y., Izumi, N., Suzuki, A., Mizuno, K. and Ohno, S. (2006) Lgl mediates apical domain disassembly by suppressing the PAR-3-aPKC-PAR-6 complex to orient apical membrane polarity. J. Cell Sci. **119**, 2107–2118

66. Yamanaka, T., Horikoshi, Y., Sugiyama, Y., Ishiyama, C., Suzuki, A., Hirose, T., Iwamatsu, A., Shinohara, A. and Ohno, S. (2003) Mammalian Lgl forms a protein complex with PAR-6 and aPKC independently of PAR-3 to regulate epithelial cell polarity. Curr. Biol. **13**, 734–743

67. Rolls, M.M., Albertson, R., Shih, H.P., Lee, C.Y. and Doe, C.Q. (2003) *Drosophila* aPKC regulates cell polarity and cell proliferation in neuroblasts and epithelia. J. Cell Biol. **163**, 1089–1098

68. Grzeschik, N.A., Parsons, L.M., Allott, M.L., Harvey, K.F. and Richardson, H.E. (2010) Lgl, aPKC, and Crumbs regulate the Salvador/Warts/Hippo pathway through two distinct mechanisms. Curr. Biol. **20**, 573–581

69. Leong, G.R., Goulding, K.R., Amin, N., Richardson, H.E. and Brumby, A.M. (2009) Scribble mutants promote aPKC and JNK-dependent epithelial neoplasia independently of Crumbs. BMC Biol. **7**, 62

70. Bilder, D., Schober, M. and Perrimon, N. (2003) Integrated activity of PDZ protein complexes regulates epithelial polarity. Nat. Cell Biol. **5**, 53–58

71. Chalmers, A.D., Pambos, M., Mason, J., Lang, S., Wylie, C. and Papalopulu, N. (2005) aPKC, Crumbs3 and Lgl2 control apicobasal polarity in early vertebrate development. Development **132**, 977–986

72. Sonawane, M., Martin-Maischein, H., Schwarz, H. and Nusslein-Volhard, C. (2009) Lgl2 and E-cadherin act antagonistically to regulate hemidesmosome formation during epidermal development in zebrafish. Development **136**, 1231–1240

73. Tanentzapf, G. and Tepass, U. (2003) Interactions between the crumbs, lethal giant larvae and bazooka pathways in epithelial polarization. Nat. Cell Biol. **5**, 46–52

74. Laprise, P. and Tepass, U. (2011) Novel insights into epithelial polarity proteins in Drosophila. Trends Cell Biol. **21**, 401–408

75. Wirtz-Peitz, F., Nishimura, T. and Knoblich, J.A. (2008) Linking cell cycle to asymmetric division: Aurora-A phosphorylates the Par complex to regulate Numb localization. Cell **135**, 161–173

76. Atwood, S.X. and Prehoda, K.E. (2009) aPKC phosphorylates Miranda to polarize fate determinants during neuroblast asymmetric cell division. Curr. Biol. **19**, 723–729

77. Siegrist, S.E. and Doe, C.Q. (2005) Microtubule-induced Pins/Galphai cortical polarity in Drosophila neuroblasts. Cell **123**, 1323–1335

78. Albertson, R. and Doe, C.Q. (2003) Dlg, Scrib and Lgl regulate neuroblast cell size and mitotic spindle asymmetry. Nat. Cell Biol. **5**, 166–170

79. Lee, C.Y., Robinson, K.J. and Doe, C.Q. (2006) Lgl, Pins and aPKC regulate neuroblast self-renewal versus differentiation. Nature **439**, 594–598

80. Peng, C.Y., Manning, L., Albertson, R. and Doe, C.Q. (2000) The tumour-suppressor genes lgl and dlg regulate basal protein targeting in Drosophila neuroblasts. Nature **408**, 596–600

81. Caussinus, E. and Gonzalez, C. (2005) Induction of tumor growth by altered stem-cell asymmetric division in Drosophila melanogaster. Nat. Genet. **37**, 1125–1129

82. Williams, S.E., Beronja, S., Pasolli, H.A. and Fuchs, E. (2011) Asymmetric cell divisions promote Notch-dependent epidermal differentiation. Nature **470**, 353–358

83. Konno, D., Shioi, G., Shitamukai, A., Mori, A., Kiyonari, H., Miyata, T. and Matsuzaki, F. (2008) Neuroepithelial progenitors undergo LGN-dependent planar divisions to maintain self-renewability during mammalian neurogenesis. Nat. Cell Biol. **10**, 93–101

84. Gray, R.S., Roszko, I. and Solnica-Krezel, L. (2011) Planar cell polarity: coordinating morphogenetic cell behaviors with embryonic polarity. Dev. Cell **21**, 120–133

85. Adler, P.N. (2002) Planar signaling and morphogenesis in Drosophila. Dev. Cell **2**, 525–535

86. Bastock, R. and Strutt, D. (2007) The planar polarity pathway promotes coordinated cell migration during Drosophila oogenesis. Development **134**, 3055–3064

87. Simons, M. and Mlodzik, M. (2008) Planar cell polarity signaling: from fly development to human disease. Annu. Rev. Genet. **42**, 517–540

88. Vladar, E.K., Antic, D. and Axelrod, J.D. (2009) Planar cell polarity signaling: the developing cell's compass. Cold Spring Harb. Perspect Biol. **1**, a002964

89. Keller, R.E., Danilchik, M., Gimlich, R. and Shih, J. (1985) The function and mechanism of convergent extension during gastrulation of Xenopus laevis. J. Embryol. Exp Morphol. **89** (Suppl.), 185–209

90. Keller, R. and Tibbetts, P. (1989) Mediolateral cell intercalation in the dorsal, axial mesoderm of Xenopus laevis. Dev. Biol. **131**, 539–549

91. Wallingford, J.B., Rowning, B.A., Vogeli, K.M., Rothbacher, U., Fraser, S.E. and Harland, R.M. (2000) Dishevelled controls cell polarity during Xenopus gastrulation. Nature **405**, 81–85

92. Rida, P.C. and Chen, P. (2009) Line up and listen: planar cell polarity regulation in the mammalian inner ear. Semin. Cell Dev. Biol. **20**, 978–985

93. Karner, C.M., Chirumamilla, R., Aoki, S., Igarashi, P., Wallingford, J.B. and Carroll, T.J. (2009) Wnt9b signaling regulates planar cell polarity and kidney tubule morphogenesis. Nat. Genet. **41**, 793–799

94. Peradziryi, H., Tolwinski, N.S. and Borchers, A. (2012) The many roles of PTK7: a versatile regulator of cell-cell communication. Arch. Biochem. Biophys., doi: 10.1016/j.abb.2011.12.019

95. Lu, X., Borchers, A.G., Jolicoeur, C., Rayburn, H., Baker, J.C. and Tessier-Lavigne, M. (2004) PTK7/CCK-4 is a novel regulator of planar cell polarity in vertebrates. Nature **430**, 93–98

96. Paudyal, A., Damrau, C., Patterson, V.L., Ermakov, A., Formstone, C., Lalanne, Z., Wells, S., Lu, X., Norris, D.P., Dean, C.H. et al. (2010) The novel mouse mutant, chuzhoi, has disruption of Ptk7 protein and exhibits defects in neural tube, heart and lung development and abnormal planar cell polarity in the ear. BMC Dev. Biol. **10**, 87

97. Montcouquiol, M., Rachel, R.A., Lanford, P.J., Copeland, N.G., Jenkins, N.A. and Kelley, M.W. (2003) Identification of Vangl2 and Scrb1 as planar polarity genes in mammals. Nature **423**, 173–177

98. Montcouquiol, M. and Kelley, M.W. (2003) Planar and vertical signals control cellular differentiation and patterning in the mammalian cochlea. J. Neurosci. **23**, 9469–9478

99. Murdoch, J.N., Rachel, R.A., Shah, S., Beermann, F., Stanier, P., Mason, C.A. and Copp, A.J. (2001) Circletail, a new mouse mutant with severe neural tube defects: chromosomal localization and interaction with the loop-tail mutation. Genomics **78**, 55–63

100. Yates, L.L., Papakrivopoulou, J., Long, D.A., Goggolidou, P., Connolly, J.O., Woolf, A.S. and Dean, C.H. (2010) The planar cell polarity gene Vangl2 is required for mammalian kidney-branching morphogenesis and glomerular maturation. Hum. Mol. Genet. **19**, 4663–4676

101. Zhan, L., Rosenberg, A., Bergami, K.C., Yu, M., Xuan, Z., Jaffe, A.B., Allred, C. and Muthuswamy, S.K. (2008) Deregulation of scribble promotes mammary tumorigenesis and reveals a role for cell polarity in carcinoma. Cell **135**, 865–878

102. Pearson, H.B., Perez-Mancera, P.A., Dow, L.E., Ryan, A., Tennstedt, P., Bogani, D., Elsum, I., Greenfield, A., Tuveson, D.A., Simon, R. and Humbert, P.O. (2011) SCRIB expression is deregulated in human prostate cancer, and its deficiency in mice promotes prostate neoplasia. J. Clin. Invest. **121**, 4257–4267

103. Djiane, A., Yogev, S. and Mlodzik, M. (2005) The apical determinants aPKC and dPatj regulate Frizzled-dependent planar cell polarity in the *Drosophila* eye. Cell **121**, 621–631

104. Caddy, J., Wilanowski, T., Darido, C., Dworkin, S., Ting, S.B., Zhao, Q., Rank, G., Auden, A., Srivastava, S., Papenfuss, T.A. et al. (2010) Epidermal wound repair is regulated by the planar cell polarity signaling pathway. Dev. Cell **19**, 138–147

105. Ludford-Menting, M.J., Oliaro, J., Sacirbegovic, F., Cheah, E.T., Pedersen, N., Thomas, S.J., Pasam, A., Iazzolino, R., Dow, L.E., Waterhouse, N.J. et al. (2005) A network of PDZ-containing proteins regulates T cell polarity and morphology during migration and immunological synapse formation. Immunity **22**, 737–748

106. Etienne-Manneville, S., Manneville, J.B., Nicholls, S., Ferenczi, M.A. and Hall, A. (2005) Cdc42 and Par6-PKCζ regulate the spatially localized association of Dlg1 and APC to control cell polarization. J. Cell Biol. **170**, 895–901

107. Etienne-Manneville, S. (2008) Polarity proteins in migration and invasion. Oncogene **27**, 6970–6980

108. Lahuna, O., Quellari, M., Achard, C., Nola, S., Meduri, G., Navarro, C., Vitale, N., Borg, J.P. and Misrahi, M. (2005) Thyrotropin receptor trafficking relies on the hScrib-βPIX-GIT1-ARF6 pathway. EMBO J. **24**, 1364–1374

109. Nola, S., Sebbagh, M., Marchetto, S., Osmani, N., Nourry, C., Audebert, S., Navarro, C., Rachel, R., Montcouquiol, M., Sans, N. et al. (2008) Scrib regulates PAK activity during the cell migration process. Hum. Mol. Genet. **17**, 3552–3565

110. Katoh, M. (2004) Identification and characterization of human GUKH2 gene *in silico*. Int. J. Oncol. **24**, 1033–1038

111. Mathew, D., Gramates, L.S., Packard, M., Thomas, U., Bilder, D., Perrimon, N., Gorczyca, M. and Budnik, V. (2002) Recruitment of scribble to the synaptic scaffolding complex requires GUK-holder, a novel DLG binding protein. Curr. Biol. **12**, 531–539

112. Brooks, S.P., Coccia, M., Tang, H.R., Kanuga, N., Machesky, L.M., Bailly, M., Cheetham, M.E. and Hardcastle, A.J. (2010) The Nance-Horan syndrome protein encodes a functional WAVE homology domain (WHD) and is important for co-ordinating actin remodelling and maintaining cell morphology. Hum. Mol. Genet. **19**, 2421–2432

113. Betschinger, J., Eisenhaber, F. and Knoblich, J.A. (2005) Phosphorylation-induced autoinhibition regulates the cytoskeletal protein Lethal (2) giant larvae. Curr. Biol. **15**, 276–282

114. Strand, D., Unger, S., Corvi, R., Hartenstein, K., Schenkel, H., Kalmes, A., Merdes, G., Neumann, B., Krieg-Schneider, F., Coy, J.F. et al. (1995) A human homologue of the *Drosophila* tumour suppressor gene l(2)gl maps to 17p11.2-12 and codes for a cytoskeletal protein that associates with nonmuscle myosin II heavy chain. Oncogene **11**, 291–301

115. Strand, D., Jakobs, R., Merdes, G., Neumann, B., Kalmes, A., Heid, H.W., Husmann, I. and Mechler, B.M. (1994) The *Drosophila* lethal(2)giant larvae tumor suppressor protein forms homo-oligomers and is associated with nonmuscle myosin II heavy chain. J. Cell Biol. **127**, 1361–1373

116. Grzeschik, N.A., Amin, N., Secombe, J., Brumby, A.M. and Richardson, H.E. (2007) Abnormalities in cell proliferation and apico-basal cell polarity are separable in *Drosophila* lgl mutant clones in the developing eye. Dev. Biol. **311**, 106–123

117. Halder, G. and Johnson, R.L. (2011) Hippo signaling: growth control and beyond. Development **138**, 9–22

118. Grzeschik, N.A., Parsons, L.M. and Richardson, H.E. (2010) Lgl, the SWH pathway and tumorigenesis: it's a matter of context & competition! Cell Cycle **16**, 3202–3212

119. Parsons, L.M., Grzeschik, N.A., Allott, M.L. and Richardson, H.E. (2010) Lgl/aPKC and Crb regulate the Salvador/Warts/Hippo pathway. Fly (Austin) **4**, 288–293

120. Enomoto, M. and Igaki, T. (2011) Deciphering tumor-suppressor signaling in flies: genetic link between Scribble/Dlg/Lgl and the Hippo pathways. J. Genet. Genomics **38**, 461–470

121. Genevet, A. and Tapon, N. (2011) The Hippo pathway and apico-basal cell polarity. Biochem. J. **436**, 213–224

122. Doggett, K., Grusche, F.A., Richardson, H.E. and Brumby, A.M. (2011) Loss of the *Drosophila* cell polarity regulator Scribbled promotes epithelial tissue overgrowth and cooperation with oncogenic Ras-Raf through impaired Hippo pathway signaling. BMC Dev. Biol. **11**, 57

123. Cordenonsi, M., Zanconato, F., Azzolin, L., Forcato, M., Rosato, A., Frasson, C., Inui, M., Montagner, M., Parenti, A.R., Poletti, A. et al. (2011) The Hippo transducer TAZ confers cancer stem cell-related traits on breast cancer cells. Cell **147**, 759–772

124. Schlegelmilch, K., Mohseni, M., Kirak, O., Pruszak, J., Rodriguez, J.R., Zhou, D., Kreger, B.T., Vasioukhin, V., Avruch, J., Brummelkamp, T.R. and Camargo, F.D. (2011) Yap1 acts downstream of α-catenin to control epidermal proliferation. Cell **144**, 782–795

125. Silvis, M.R., Kreger, B.T., Lien, W.H., Klezovitch, O., Rudakova, G.M., Camargo, F.D., Lantz, D.M., Seykora, J.T. and Vasioukhin, V. (2011) α-Catenin is a tumor suppressor that controls cell accumulation by regulating the localization and activity of the transcriptional coactivator Yap1. Sci. Signaling **4**, ra33

126. Fernandez, B.G., Gaspar, P., Bras-Pereira, C., Jezowska, B., Rebelo, S.R. and Janody, F. (2011) Actin-capping protein and the Hippo pathway regulate F-actin and tissue growth in *Drosophila*. Development **138**, 2337–2346

127. Sansores-Garcia, L., Bossuyt, W., Wada, K., Yonemura, S., Tao, C., Sasaki, H. and Halder, G. (2011) Modulating F-actin organization induces organ growth by affecting the Hippo pathway. EMBO J. **30**, 2325–2335

128. Skouloudaki, K., Puetz, M., Simons, M., Courbard, J.R., Boehlke, C., Hartleben, B., Engel, C., Moeller, M.J., Englert, C., Bollig, F. et al. (2009) Scribble participates in Hippo signaling and is required for normal zebrafish pronephros development. Proc. Natl. Acad. Sci. U.S.A. **106**, 8579–8584

129. Nagasaka, K., Pim, D., Massimi, P., Thomas, M., Tomaic, V., Subbaiah, V.K., Kranjec, C., Nakagawa, S., Yano, T., Taketani, Y. et al. (2010) The cell polarity regulator hScrib controls ERK activation through a KIM site-dependent interaction. Oncogene **29**, 5311–5321

130. Kern, F., Niault, T. and Baccarini, M. (2011) Ras and Raf pathways in epidermis development and carcinogenesis. Br. J. Cancer **104**, 229–234

131. Zeniou-Meyer, M., Liu, Y., Begle, A., Olanich, M.E., Hanauer, A., Becherer, U., Rettig, J., Bader, M.F. and Vitale, N. (2008) The Coffin-Lowry syndrome-associated protein RSK2 is implicated in calcium-regulated exocytosis through the regulation of PLD1. Proc. Natl. Acad. Sci. U.S.A. **105**, 8434–8439

132. Yin, G., Haendeler, J., Yan, C. and Berk, B.C. (2004) GIT1 functions as a scaffold for MEK1-extracellular signal-regulated kinase 1 and 2 activation by angiotensin II and epidermal growth factor. Mol. Cell. Biol. **24**, 875–885

133. Audebert, S., Navarro, C., Nourry, C., Chasserot-Golaz, S., Lecine, P., Bellaiche, Y., Dupont, J.L., Premont, R.T., Sempere, C., Strub, J.M. et al. (2004) Mammalian Scribble forms a tight complex with the βPIX exchange factor. Curr. Biol. **14**, 987–995

134. Reischauer, S., Levesque, M.P., Nusslein-Volhard, C. and Sonawane, M. (2009) Lgl2 executes its function as a tumor suppressor by regulating ErbB signaling in the zebrafish epidermis. PLoS Genet. **5**, e1000720

135. Rivard, N. (2009) Phosphatidylinositol 3-kinase: a key regulator in adherens junction formation and function. Front. Biosci. **14**, 510–522

136. Chalhoub, N. and Baker, S.J. (2009) PTEN and the PI3-kinase pathway in cancer. Annu. Rev. Pathol. **4**, 127–150

137. Adey, N.B., Huang, L., Ormonde, P.A., Baumgard, M.L., Pero, R., Byreddy, D.V., Tavtigian, S.V. and Bartel, P.L. (2000) Threonine phosphorylation of the MMAC1/PTEN PDZ binding domain both inhibits and stimulates PDZ binding. Cancer Res. **60**, 35–37

138. Frese, K.K., Latorre, I.J., Chung, S.H., Caruana, G., Bernstein, A., Jones, S.N., Donehower, L.A., Justice, M.J., Garner, C.C. and Javier, R.T. (2006) Oncogenic function for the Dlg1 mammalian homolog of the *Drosophila* discs-large tumor suppressor. EMBO J. **25**, 1406–1417

139. Willecke, M., Toggweiler, J. and Basler, K. (2011) Loss of PI3K blocks cell-cycle progression in a *Drosophila* tumor model. Oncogene **30**, 4067–4074

140. Li, X., Yang, H., Liu, J., Schmidt, M.D. and Gao, T. (2011) Scribble-mediated membrane targeting of PHLPP1 is required for its negative regulation of Akt. EMBO Rep. **12**, 818–824

141. Lu, H. and Bilder, D. (2005) Endocytic control of epithelial polarity and proliferation in *Drosophila*. Nat. Cell Biol. **7**, 1232–1239

142. Shivas, J.M., Morrison, H.A., Bilder, D. and Skop, A.R. (2010) Polarity and endocytosis: reciprocal regulation. Trends Cell Biol. **20**, 445–452

143. Balklava, Z., Pant, S., Fares, H. and Grant, B.D. (2007) Genome-wide analysis identifies a general requirement for polarity proteins in endocytic traffic. Nat. Cell Biol. **9**, 1066–1073

144. Leibfried, A., Fricke, R., Morgan, M.J., Bogdan, S. and Bellaiche, Y. (2008) *Drosophila* Cip4 and WASp define a branch of the Cdc42-Par6-aPKC pathway regulating E-cadherin endocytosis. Curr. Biol. **18**, 1639–1648

145. Georgiou, M., Marinari, E., Burden, J. and Baum, B. (2008) Cdc42, Par6, and aPKC regulate Arp2/3-mediated endocytosis to control local adherens junction stability. Curr. Biol. **18**, 1631–1638

146. Harris, K.P. and Tepass, U. (2008) Cdc42 and Par proteins stabilize dynamic adherens junctions in the *Drosophila* neuroectoderm through regulation of apical endocytosis. J. Cell Biol. **183**, 1129–1143

147. He, B. and Guo, W. (2009) The exocyst complex in polarized exocytosis. Curr. Opin. Cell Biol. **21**, 537–542

148. Blankenship, J.T., Fuller, M.T. and Zallen, J.A. (2007) The *Drosophila* homolog of the Exo84 exocyst subunit promotes apical epithelial identity. J. Cell Sci. **120**, 3099–3110

149. Musch, A., Cohen, D., Yeaman, C., Nelson, W.J., Rodriguez-Boulan, E. and Brennwald, P.J. (2002) Mammalian homolog of *Drosophila* tumor suppressor lethal (2) giant larvae interacts with basolateral exocytic machinery in Madin-Darby canine kidney cells. Mol. Biol. Cell **13**, 158–168

150. Gangar, A., Rossi, G., Andreeva, A., Hales, R. and Brennwald, P. (2005) Structurally conserved interaction of Lgl family with SNAREs is critical to their cellular function. Curr. Biol. **15**, 1136–1142

151. Zhang, X., Wang, P., Gangar, A., Zhang, J., Brennwald, P., TerBush, D. and Guo, W. (2005) Lethal giant larvae proteins interact with the exocyst complex and are involved in polarized exocytosis. J. Cell Biol. **170**, 273–283

152. Massimi, P., Narayan, N., Thomas, M., Gammoh, N., Strand, S., Strand, D. and Banks, L. (2008) Regulation of the hDlg/hScrib/Hugl-1 tumour suppressor complex. Exp. Cell Res. **314**, 3306–3317

153. Wang, T., Liu, Y., Xu, X.H., Deng, C.Y., Wu, K.Y., Zhu, J., Fu, X.Q., He, M. and Luo, Z.G. (2011) Lgl1 activation of rab10 promotes axonal membrane trafficking underlying neuronal polarization. Dev. Cell **21**, 431–444

154. Giebel, B. and Wodarz, A. (2006) Tumor suppressors: control of signaling by endocytosis. Curr. Biol. **16**, R91–R92

155. Thomas, M., Narayan, N., Pim, D., Tomaic, V., Massimi, P., Nagasaka, K., Kranjec, C., Gammoh, N. and Banks, L. (2008) Human papillomaviruses, cervical cancer and cell polarity. Oncogene **27**, 7018–7030

156. Gardiol, D., Kuhne, C., Glaunsinger, B., Lee, S.S., Javier, R. and Banks, L. (1999) Oncogenic human papillomavirus E6 proteins target the discs large tumour suppressor for proteasome-mediated degradation. Oncogene **18**, 5487–5496

157. Glaunsinger, B.A., Lee, S.S., Thomas, M., Banks, L. and Javier, R. (2000) Interactions of the PDZ-protein MAGI-1 with adenovirus E4-ORF1 and high-risk papillomavirus E6 oncoproteins. Oncogene **19**, 5270–5280

158. Lee, S.S., Glaunsinger, B., Mantovani, F., Banks, L. and Javier, R.T. (2000) Multi-PDZ domain protein MUPP1 is a cellular target for both adenovirus E4-ORF1 and high-risk papillomavirus type 18 E6 oncoproteins. J. Virol. **74**, 9680–9693

159. Nakagawa, S. and Huibregtse, J.M. (2000) Human scribble (Vartul) is targeted for ubiquitin-mediated degradation by the high-risk papillomavirus E6 proteins and the E6AP ubiquitin-protein ligase. Mol. Cell. Biol. **20**, 8244–8253

160. Kiyono, T., Hiraiwa, A., Fujita, M., Hayashi, Y., Akiyama, T. and Ishibashi, M. (1997) Binding of high-risk human papillomavirus E6 oncoproteins to the human homologue of the *Drosophila* discs large tumor suppressor protein. Proc. Natl. Acad. Sci. U.S.A. **94**, 11612–11616

161. Glaunsinger, B.A., Weiss, R.S., Lee, S.S. and Javier, R. (2001) Link of the unique oncogenic properties of adenovirus type 9 E4-ORF1 to a select interaction with the candidate tumor suppressor protein ZO-2. EMBO J. **20**, 5578–5586

162. Lee, S.S., Weiss, R.S. and Javier, R.T. (1997) Binding of human virus oncoproteins to hDlg/SAP97, a mammalian homolog of the *Drosophila* discs large tumor suppressor protein. Proc. Natl. Acad. Sci. U.S.A. **94**, 6670–6675

163. Okajima, M., Takahashi, M., Higuchi, M., Ohsawa, T., Yoshida, S., Yoshida, Y., Oie, M., Tanaka, Y., Gejyo, F. and Fujii, M. (2008) Human T-cell leukemia virus type 1 Tax induces an aberrant clustering of the tumor suppressor Scribble through the PDZ domain-binding motif dependent and independent interaction. Virus Genes **37**, 231–240

164. Javier, R.T. (2008) Cell polarity proteins: common targets for tumorigenic human viruses. Oncogene **27**, 7031–7046

165. Huang, L. and Muthuswamy, S.K. (2010) Polarity protein alterations in carcinoma: a focus on emerging roles for polarity regulators. Curr. Opin. Genet. Dev. **20**, 41–50

166. Gardiol, D., Zacchi, A., Petrera, F., Stanta, G. and Banks, L. (2006) Human discs large and scrib are localized at the same regions in colon mucosa and changes in their expression patterns are correlated with loss of tissue architecture during malignant progression. Int. J. Cancer **119**, 1285–1290

167. Lin, H.T., Steller, M.A., Aish, L., Hanada, T. and Chishti, A.H. (2004) Differential expression of human Dlg in cervical intraepithelial neoplasias. Gynecol. Oncol. **93**, 422–428

168. Lisovsky, M., Dresser, K., Baker, S., Fisher, A., Woda, B., Banner, B. and Lauwers, G.Y. (2009) Cell polarity protein Lgl2 is lost or aberrantly localized in gastric dysplasia and adenocarcinoma: an immunohistochemical study. Mod. Pathol. **22**, 977–984

169. Grifoni, D., Garoia, F., Schimanski, C.C., Schmitz, G., Laurenti, E., Galle, P.R., Pession, A., Cavicchi, S. and Strand, D. (2004) The human protein Hugl-1 substitutes for *Drosophila* lethal giant larvae tumour suppressor function *in vivo*. Oncogene **23**, 8688–8694

170. Nakagawa, S., Yano, T., Nakagawa, K., Takizawa, S., Suzuki, Y., Yasugi, T., Huibregtse, J.M. and Taketani, Y. (2004) Analysis of the expression and localisation of a LAP protein, human scribble, in the normal and neoplastic epithelium of uterine cervix. Br. J. Cancer **90**, 194–199

171. Ouyang, Z., Zhan, W. and Dan, L. (2010) hScrib, a human homolog of *Drosophila* neoplastic tumor suppressor, is involved in the progress of endometrial cancer. Oncol. Res. **18**, 593–599

172. Vaira, V., Faversani, A., Dohi, T., Maggioni, M., Nosotti, M., Tosi, D., Altieri, D.C. and Bosari, S. (2011) Aberrant overexpression of the cell polarity module scribble in human cancer. Am. J. Pathol. **178**, 2478–2483

173. Nolan, M.E., Aranda, V., Lee, S., Lakshmi, B., Basu, S., Allred, D.C. and Muthuswamy, S.K. (2008) The polarity protein Par6 induces cell proliferation and is overexpressed in breast cancer. Cancer Res. **68**, 8201–8209

174. Viloria-Petit, A.M., David, L., Jia, J.Y., Erdemir, T., Bane, A.L., Pinnaduwage, D., Roncari, L., Narimatsu, M., Bose, R., Moffat, J. et al. (2009) A role for the TGFβ-Par6 polarity pathway in breast cancer progression. Proc. Natl. Acad. Sci. U.S.A. **106**, 14028–14033

175. Zen, K., Yasui, K., Gen, Y., Dohi, O., Wakabayashi, N., Mitsufuji, S., Itoh, Y., Zen, Y., Nakanuma, Y., Taniwaki, M. et al. (2009) Defective expression of polarity protein PAR-3 gene (PARD3) in esophageal squamous cell carcinoma. Oncogene **28**, 2910–2918

176. Grifoni, D., Garoia, F., Bellosta, P., Parisi, F., De Biase, D., Collina, G., Strand, D., Cavicchi, S. and Pession, A. (2007) aPKCζ cortical loading is associated with Lgl cytoplasmic release and tumor growth in *Drosophila* and human epithelia. Oncogene **26**, 5960–5965

177. Karp, C.M., Tan, T.T., Mathew, R., Nelson, D., Mukherjee, C., Degenhardt, K., Karantza-Wadsworth, V. and White, E. (2008) Role of the polarity determinant crumbs in suppressing mammalian epithelial tumor progression. Cancer Res. **68**, 4105–4115

178. Kuphal, S., Wallner, S., Schimanski, C.C., Bataille, F., Hofer, P., Strand, S., Strand, D. and Bosserhoff, A.K. (2006) Expression of Hugl-1 is strongly reduced in malignant melanoma. Oncogene **25**, 103–110

179. Schimanski, C.C., Schmitz, G., Kashyap, A., Bosserhoff, A.K., Bataille, F., Schafer, S.C., Lehr, H.A., Berger, M.R., Galle, P.R., Strand, S. and Strand, D. (2005) Reduced expression of Hugl-1, the human homologue of *Drosophila* tumour suppressor gene lgl, contributes to progression of colorectal cancer. Oncogene **24**, 3100–3109

180. Brumby, A.M. and Richardson, H.E. (2003) Scribble mutants cooperate with oncogenic Ras or Notch to cause neoplastic overgrowth in *Drosophila*. EMBO J. **22**, 5769–5779

181. Froldi, F., Ziosi, M., Garoia, F., Pession, A., Grzeschik, N.A., Bellosta, P., Strand, D., Richardson, H.E. and Grifoni, D. (2010) The lethal giant larvae tumour suppressor mutation requires dMyc oncoprotein to promote clonal malignancy. BMC Biol. **8**, 33

Index

O

occludin, 42, 44, 45, 46, 47, 48, 49, 50, 84, 87, 142

P

p120-catenin, 83, 84

PAR, 1, 3, 4, 5, 6, 7, 8, 9, 10, 16, 22, 23, 24, 61, 62, 63, 64, 65, 84, 89, 90, 96, 97, 100, 102, 103, 104, 105, 132, 133, 134, 147, 153

PARtitioning defective (see PAR)

PCP, 142, 146, 149, 151, 152, 153, 159

PDZ domain, 4, 88, 122, 123, 143, 144, 145, 147, 157

PH domain, 20

phosphatase and tensin homologue deleted on chromosome 10 (see PTEN)

phosphoinositide, 15–25, 34, 48, 60, 115, 131, 132, 155

phosphoinositide 3-kinase (see PI3K)

PI3K, 18, 20, 21, 22, 23, 24, 34, 60, 61, 63, 64, 65, 115, 131, 132, 155

PIKfyve, 48, 49

planar cell polarity (see PCP)

plasma membrane, 15–25, 29, 30, 31, 36, 37, 41, 43, 44, 45, 46, 47, 48, 49, 96, 99, 117, 146, 147, 155, 156

pleckstrin homology domain (see PH domain)

polarity
    establishment, 1, 2, 5, 9, 10
    maintenance, 7, 103

primary cilium, 30

progenitor, 71, 79, 97, 98, 99, 100, 101, 104, 105, 106

PTEN, 16, 18, 20, 21, 22, 23, 24, 60, 136, 155

R

Rab, 13, 33, 49, 50

Rab GTPase, 62

Ras GTPase, 63, 155

RE, 29, 30, 31, 32, 33, 34, 35, 36, 37, 47

recycling endosome (see RE)

Rho GTPase, 21, 22, 63, 89, 90, 116, 151, 153

S

SAD kinase, 61, 62

SARAH domain, 120, 121, 122

Sav1, 112, 113, 114, 121, 122

Scribble, 88, 96, 97, 102, 103, 134, 141, 142, 143, 144, 145, 146, 148, 151, 152, 153, 154, 155, 156, 157, 158, 159

senescence, 69, 70, 73, 74, 76, 77, 79

septate junction, 96, 130, 132, 134, 148

spindle positioning, 3, 10, 62

stem cell, 10, 70, 71, 76, 78, 86, 88, 97, 98, 99, 101, 105, 106, 111–124, 146, 147, 154

symmetric division, 102, 149

symplekin, 86, 87

synapses of the amphid defective kinase (see SAD kinase)

T

TAZ, 88, 90, 111, 112, 113, 114, 115, 116, 117, 118, 119, 121, 122, 123, 154

TGFβ, 72, 90, 115, 116, 117, 123, 133

tight junction, 17, 24, 30, 41–50, 84, 96, 113, 123, 130, 142, 146, 148

transcriptional coactivator with PDZ-binding motif (see TAZ)

transcytosis, 34, 35, 43

transforming growth factor β (see TGFβ)

U

ubiquitin, 46, 119, 123

V

vesicle trafficking, 145, 156, 158

W

WW domain, 117, 119, 121

Y

YAP, 83, 85, 86, 88–89, 90, 91, 111, 112, 113, 114, 115, 116, 117, 118, 119, 120, 121, 122, 123, 154

Yes-associated protein (see YAP)